Dancing Through Cancer

by Laurie Riddell Geary

Cancer Survivor and Dancer Extraordinaire

Order from
Amazon. com

Copyright © 2013 by Laurie R. Geary

Table of Contents

Dedication

To my sons: *Scott* and *Derek,*
and my grandchildren:
Madison, Taylor, and *Jack,*
my most important legacies.

Note to Reader

The facts and statistics about lung cancer that I share in this book are figures I learned through my readings and through conferences I attended – sources that I believe to be reliable. I am not a lung cancer expert; I am a cancer patient, survivor, and an advocate. My description of medical procedures and my understanding of the biology of cancer are as a layman. I believe my posts are fundamentally correct, but to the extent they are not, only I am to blame.

Introduction

In this book I share my cancer journey – what it's like to live with Stage IV lung cancer and what I'm doing to enjoy my life despite that reality. My life changed completely when I got my diagnosis. Suddenly my priorities were rearranged; I realized that what matters most to me now are my family and friends – nothing else is important. And all that *really* matters is love – my love for them and their love for me.

The motivation to write a blog came shortly after my surprise diagnosis in 2008. My first reaction had been, "Oh no! My three grandchildren will never get to know me." They were relatively young then (ages 13, 11, and 6), and I didn't feel we had shared enough time together. I want them to know me as an active, fun grandmother, someone who will ski or swim or sail or hike or bike or dance with them. I want them to know my values and my life-long learnings; I want to share in their significant events; I want to know about their dreams and desires; I want to be a great-grandmother! I want to share in their lives for many more years! I was afraid they would only remember me as a sickly cancer victim.

They lived in Massachusetts for five wonderful years; we shared some special times together. I was fortunate to be able to recuperate from lung surgery and chemotherapy at their house. Sadly, they moved back to California shortly thereafter. Now they are teenagers preoccupied with their lives. I see them rarely and, when I do, they are busy with school, friends, sports, and other activities. I fear they will never know me the way I would want. So I am writing this in the hopes that someday they may read it and get to know me a little better. It's my legacy to them.

This blog – now book – has taken on a bigger purpose, however. Once I started writing it I realized it might be helpful to other cancer patients and their loved ones. And now I think my book will help *anyone* learn ways to prevent cancer. As I write about what has helped me live a meaningful and happy life despite my cancer treatments, I hope that what has helped me will help others. I include resources – books, films, and websites – along with recommendations of ways to live peacefully with a life-threatening cancer diagnosis. I trust that others will benefit from all that I have learned and experienced. It's my way of leaving a legacy to others as well. I want to feel that my little time on this earth has made a positive difference in the lives of others.

In this book I share with you all the (shocking) lung cancer facts I have learned. There are numerous posts on nutrition espousing the importance of eating a plant-based, sugar-free diet for prevention and healing. I discuss stress management, risk-taking, alternative healing modalities, and the importance of living in a healing environment. I share my experiences dealing with medical/surgical treatments, and managing medication side effects. I also share my fears and challenges, my feelings and values. I offer my learnings and "coachable moments." I delve into my spiritual quest and share my thoughts on death and dying. I acknowledge my wonderful support system and how important they are in helping me get through it all. Mostly I explain why and how I am *Dancing Through Cancer*.

The posts in this book are not in the chronological order they were in my blog. I have organized the posts in a structure that makes more sense, one that is more cohesive and thematic. So at times a post may seem out of sync, and there are redundancies – statistics mentioned frequently, resources mentioned more than once, key points and quotes repeatedly made – but these are meant to reinforce the importance of the information.

At the five-year mark of my cancer diagnosis, I celebrate "beating the odds" since most Stage IV lung cancer patients don't survive more than two years after diagnosis. Only 5% of lung cancer patients reach the 5-year mark; I've reached it! Ta Da! Everything points to my living a few more years; I plan to make the most of those years!

My blog (www.ingearcoaching.com/blog) will continue (and I hope you will continue to read it), but for now I give you this book to peruse and enjoy. I hope it helps you or someone you know in some small way.

My Story

"You have lung cancer." My surgeon had just called to tell me this after reading my chest x-ray taken in preparation for a scheduled breast lumpectomy. I remember standing all alone in my condo holding the phone, in shock, having my first out-of-body experience, thinking *this isn't real, this isn't happening to me!* I am a non-smoker, there was no family history of lung cancer, and I had always lived a healthy lifestyle (I thought). I immediately got on the phone and started calling my family and close friends who reacted in the same shocked way. And then they started taking care of me, as they continue to care for me now. I couldn't manage this journey without them.

It all started in March, 2008, when I went in for a routine mammogram (that I had been putting off for months) and was horrified to be told that I had breast cancer (DCIS: Ductal Carcinoma in Situ). But the news got worse: the chest x-ray I needed in preparation for the lumpectomy to remove the small breast tumor found cancer in my right lung!

The next few weeks consisted of a whirlwind of tests (bronchoscopy, PET scan, cat scan, MRI, endless blood work, etc.) leading to the decision to remove the top lobe of my right lung (where there was a large tumor) and a section of my right lower lobe (where there was another smaller, different tumor). Meanwhile, the lumpectomy was postponed. The good news was that none of the three tumors was related; all were different cancers (these are called *synchrous* tumors: tumors that are independent of each other). This meant that the cancer hadn't metastasized throughout my body. They called it Stage II-B at that point.

In June I had lung surgery – a *lobectomy*. Unfortunately, cancer was found in my *mediastinum* lymph glands (in my throat), which meant it had metastasized. I was "upgraded" to Stage III-A.

Recovery from surgery was awful. I was in the hospital for a week, learning how to breathe again. I remember saying to someone that I would rather kill myself than go through that again! Many friends and family visited me, although I was always in a fog of pain and discomfort.

My son, Scott, and wife, Lisa, (and grandchildren: Madison, Taylor, and Jack) took me into their home (and even gave me *their* bed so I could be closer to all the family activities). They took care of me for two months while I slowly recuperated. This was not a fun period of time, but it was very special to be in their loving and supportive care. My friends made a caravan to their house bringing me all their love and support too. Slowly I healed.

The next plan was for breast surgery, then chemotherapy, and targeted chest radiation.

After recovering from lung surgery (around six weeks) I had a breast *lumpectomy*, which went smoothly. I was told I had a 99% chance of recovery, so I wasn't concerned about the breast cancer; it's the lung cancer that worried me.

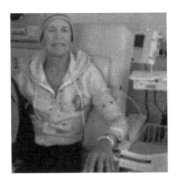

Getting an Infusion

Next was chemotherapy: four sessions – sitting one whole day in the chair having a chemical infusion into my arm – then three weeks off to recuperate. The side effects were cumulative, so after each session I got sicker and sicker.

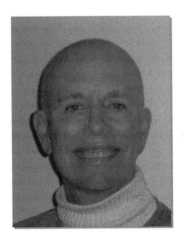

My Bald Look

Of course, I lost my hair immediately. However, I quickly realized how insignificant losing my hair was compared to all the other unpleasant side effects (nausea, lack of appetite, mouth sores, fatigue, constipation, etc.). I've learned to love my new short hairdo, and that says a lot from someone who had the same long blonde hairstyle her entire life (see "It's Not About the Hair...").

My friends and family were amazingly supportive during this whole process; they just stepped in and took care of me. One friend organized everything to make sure someone always went with me to my doctor appointments and chemotherapy sessions; she also arranged for me to stay with someone each weekend after chemotherapy when the side effects tended to be the worst. Scheduling really helped.

My two sons and daughter-in-law and grandchildren also devoted their time to caring for me. I practically lived at my older son's house for six months, and later my younger son came to care for me in my condo (earlier, he even camped out in the hospital with me). I was never alone; I felt surrounded by love and support, which made a positive difference in my healing, I'm sure.

By January, 2009, I was ready for targeted radiation therapy: 35 sessions, one every day for six weeks. I was fortunate that my condo was only a 10-minute walk to Mass General Hospital, so I walked over there every day. The radiation was painless – a piece-of-cake compared to chemotherapy. However, I did develop such a nasty rash on my chest they had to stop treatments for a week (which shows how strong those rays are). But I finished by March, when I took advantage of my freedom and new-found energy and joined my nephew and his wife in Aspen to ski.

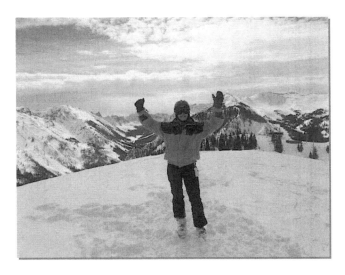

Skiing in Aspen after Treatments

After that, I had follow-up cat scans every three months, and for a long while the scans were clear. Then there was surprisingly bad news during my appointment in January, 2010.

"You now have tumors in both lungs and a metastasis to your brain." I was speechless, horrified, shocked! I was so confident that I was cured that I had gone to this appointment alone. (Never again! A friend always goes with me to my doctor appointments now.) Since ending radiation in March, the cat scans had all been clear; I thought I was home free. But, I have since learned there is a "blood-brain barrier" while undergoing chemotherapy, thus none of the chemicals can get into the brain. So the cancer seeks an escape route, and the unprotected brain is an easy target.

Now, the lung cancer had clearly metastasized into my brain and probably throughout my body. I was upgraded to Stage IV: un-curable lung cancer. It was devastating news.

But I had no time to feel sorry for myself or be immobilized by depression. I immediately had a procedure that shoots radiation beams into the brain, targeted directly at the tumor.

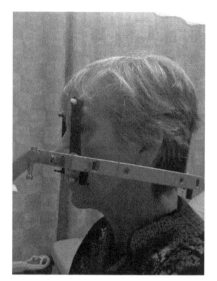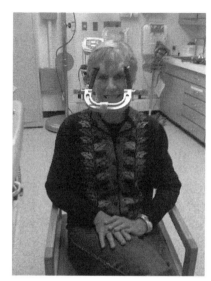

Stereotactic Radio Surgery

Called SRS or Stereotactic RadioSurgery, a metal halo is screwed into the skull in four places, and then the halo is screwed to the table (stability is important). A good friend, a former nurse practitioner, flew up from Georgia to support me through all this. The procedure itself was painless (and successful); the screws in the head are what hurt. Then for months I had a numb section on the top of my head and, for years now, it has become an itchy section.

After SRS, I started taking Tarceva® (Erlotinib) the miracle chemotherapy pill that has been very effective in reducing tumors in patients, like me, who have the mutated gene, EGFR (Epidermal Growth Factor Receptor). Non-smokers and women typically get the EGFR mutation, but we don't understand why (see "Tarceva® Trials and Tribulations"). Tarceva® is able to permeate the blood-brain barrier; my brain is protected!

Currently – April, 2013 – I have taken the pill every day for over three years and each cat scan (every three months) has shown the tumors shrinking and disappearing! I now only have one MRI per year to check my brain for tumors since they are so sure nothing is there any longer. I don't even think about the breast cancer; I have yearly mammograms and all is well there.

There will come a time when Tarceva® stops working (average effectiveness is two years). I am beating the average so far, and am hopeful that I still have many more years with its effectiveness. Then I'm counting on a new drug to be discovered when the time comes.

The side effects of the pill aren't pleasant (I've counted over 25 different effects so far (see "Managing Medication Side Effects"). However, the side effects are tolerable; I've learned to live with them. And, of course, they're better than the alternative!

I'm fortunate that I have a lot of energy and basically feel pretty well, so I can focus on living my life and enjoying each and every day. I'm one of the lucky ones whose quality of life is not too badly impacted by the medication and treatments. But I hold my breath every time I have another cat scan; I'm always anxious until I hear the results – I have *scanxiety!* But I hold onto my optimism and hope.

I will always have lung cancer; I will never be cancer-free. I will most likely die of lung cancer, sooner than later. I live with the scary statistic that only 5% of lung cancer patients live past five years. I'm in unchartered territory.

All I can do is make the most of my situation and live my life – each day – as best I can. I share with you how I am now living my life – a life that is actually much richer and more meaningful than it has ever been. *I'm dancing through cancer* as positively as I can. I can choose to focus on what's wrong with my life – the negative – or I can choose to focus on what's right with my life – the positive. I choose positive!

Attitude is everything!

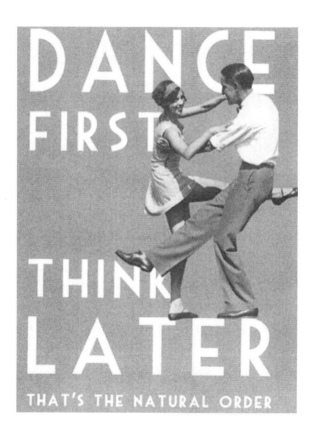

Lung Cancer

Facts and Information
(What I've Learned So Far)

Recent Advances in Lung Cancer Research: March, 2013

The National Lung Cancer Partnership just sponsored a webinar given by Dr. David Spigel, Director of Lung Cancer Research at Sarah Cannon Research Institute. The webinar is well worth watching if you have an hour's time (www.lungcancerpartnership.org). Meanwhile, I will share the key information here.

I felt very optimistic and hopeful after watching this webinar. Cancer (including lung cancer) research is the most advanced it has ever been; it's a "whole new ball game," as they say. In the past, all cancers were treated the same way: a "one size fits all" approach where the same chemotherapy was used for all. Treatment was like throwing stuff on a wall to see what sticks. Now, "Molecular Profiling" has changed the landscape of oncology. By understanding the molecular features of lung cancer, treatment can be personalized.

Recent research has shown that not all lung cancers are the same. There are four main types: Non Small Cell Adenocarcinoma (NSCLC), Squamous Cell, Small Cell, and

Large Cell. NSCLC, the largest type, makes up 62% of all lung cancers, and within that type different mutations have been identified (23 mutations so far). The main mutations are KRAS (32%), EGFR (23%), ALK (3%), and Her2 (3%); 36% of mutations are unknown. These are called "driver mutations" because each one "drives" a different type of lung cancer. What's important about this is that each mutation responds to a different chemo drug; thus, treatment can be specialized.

Another key discovery: mutations appear to be mutually exclusive. People are unlikely to get a different mutation once they have one.

I am EGFR positive and have been taking the chemo pill, Tarceva®, known to be effective with the EGFR mutation. In fact, for people who are EGFR positive, studies showed that Tarceva® worked better than chemotherapy. This drug has worked *very* effectively for me for over three years, and I'm optimistic that it will keep on working for a few more years.

Unfortunately, cancer always figures out a way around any chemotherapy, so I'm worried about what I will do when that happens. I was glad to find out that there are two chemo pills (called "next generation EGFR inhibitors") already available, Afatinib and MedMAB, which have proven to be as effective as Tarceva® (although neither is FDA approved yet). Of course, dealing with the new side effects is always a concern, but I'll cross that bridge when I come to it.

Other advances in lung cancer research mentioned include …

…better screening for lung cancer (now there will be automatic testing for EGFR and ALK since they are so common).

...faster time in getting chemo drugs FDA approved and into the market.

...improved technology to help with research advances.

...immunotherapy: finding ways to thwart cancer from "tricking" the immune system.

...better awareness of lung cancer, leading to more successful fundraising for research.

...offering better palliative care, which has been proven to extend survival.

I was surprised and pleased that *my* oncologist, Jennifer Temel, was acknowledged for her important research on palliative care, which includes...

...education, clarification, and understanding of treatment goals.

...symptom management of pain, mood, gastrointestinal and pulmonary issues.

...help with decision-making.

...help with coping strategies.

Lung cancer awareness is growing; more voices are speaking up! More and more websites and blogs are sprouting. There is more research, and research does pay off! The *Free to Breathe* organization sponsors fundraisers for lung cancer research. *The National Lung Cancer Partnership* annually awards "Young Investigator Grants" for lung cancer research. They also sponsor an annual *Lung Cancer Advocacy Summit* (which I attended) where hundreds of lung cancer survivors and people touched by lung cancer are trained and supported to advocate for lung cancer. This blog/book is part of my advocacy; I hope you will join the voices! Our Goal - **Beat Lung Cancer**!

Visit www.nationallungcancerpartnership.org/shop/free-resources.html and watch the webinar to see all the charts and studies.

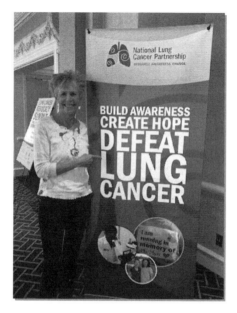

At the National Lung Cancer Partnership Conference

Some Interesting, Mostly Unknown Facts About Cancer

Every person has cancer cells in their body; cancer cells occur between six to more than ten times in a person's lifetime. When the person's immune system is strong the cancer cells are destroyed; when their immune system is weak, the cancer will grow. Our immune system gets weakened when we age, when we have nutritional deficiencies, when we smoke, when we're stressed, when we're exposed to environmental toxins, etc. Lung cancer is one of the deadliest forms of cancer because it is rarely detected early.

Lung cancer is the single biggest killer among cancers, responsible for nearly 30% of all cancer deaths. The incidence of lung cancer has *increased* six-fold over the last 30 years. The survival rate for lung cancer has hardly changed since the war on cancer began in 1971, yet there are fewer research dollars devoted to lung cancer than any other major cancer group. There are 220,000 new cases of lung cancer diagnosed each year, and 160,000 people will die of it. In the next five years 800,000 people will die of lung cancer. Lung cancer mortality has dramatically risen in women, particularly older women, and it is still rising. Between 1970 and 1994, lung cancer deaths among women over 55 increased by 400%, more than the rise in the rates of breast and colon and prostate cancer combined.

One in 31,000 golfers will make a hole-in-one; one in three people will be diagnosed with cancer.

Did you know these facts about lung cancer? Most people are shocked to hear this information. There is such a hue and cry about breast cancer, with lots of marches and other fundraising events. Why aren't there more marches and fundraisers for lung cancer research? I think much of the reason is due to the stigma of lung cancer, i.e. the belief that lung cancer victims deserve what they got because of smoking. And smokers with lung cancer tend to live with feelings of guilt, so they don't speak up. Lung cancer is seen as a self-inflicted disease, not really worthy of public research funding.

Blaming smokers for lung cancer is a big factor in keeping funding for research away. The belief being that if smoking causes lung cancer, then *just stop smoking*; if you smoke you deserve the consequences. But if a smoker gets lung cancer, do they really deserve to be blamed? Remember how cigarettes were part of the "mess kit" for soldiers in WWII? And how advertising from the tobacco companies made smoking attractive and sexy? Thousands became addicted to nicotine before they knew the dangers. It took years of multiple lawsuits to stop the advertising. Now, with education, there are fewer smokers – but lung cancer is still rising!

The American Cancer Society's solution to the lung cancer epidemic is to urge people to quit smoking; this is such a dangerous misperception.

Most people don't know that 15% of people with lung cancer are non-smokers; 40% of non-smokers and former smokers *combined* will get lung cancer this year. These statistics contradict the universal belief that lung cancer is only caused by smoking. The reality is that more and more non-smokers are getting lung cancer, and we don't really know why.

Because of the loud voices raising awareness about breast cancer there has been a lot more funding for breast cancer research, which has been very effective: now 85% of women with breast cancer survive. Funding for lung cancer is still miniscule; it is the least funded of all the cancers. Only 15% of lung cancer patients survive, so how can they have much of a voice?

I sometimes think it's just the luck of the draw who gets cancer and who doesn't. We still don't understand why some people get cancer and some don't. If you have cancer, you certainly didn't deserve to get it, and I'm sure you are doing what you can to be healthier: eating right, exercising, getting support from your friends, and avoiding stress. If you don't have cancer, I hope my information will inspire you to do everything you can to prevent it from occurring in your body. Prevention is much easier than management! This entire book is meant to give you the information you need to prevent or manage cancer.

November is National Lung Cancer Awareness Month

Did you know that November is Lung Cancer Awareness Month? Probably not. But why not? Most likely because you believe that lung cancer is caused by smoking, therefore, if you don't smoke or aren't around smoke, you're safe, right? WRONG!

Forty percent of people who don't smoke (or who quit smoking) get cancer! Actually, if you have lungs you can get lung cancer! Did you know that:

- Cancer is the second leading cause of death for both men and women and lung cancer is the #1 cancer killer!

- Lung cancer is responsible for more cancer deaths than breast, colon, and prostate cancer combined! Yet funding for lung cancer research is the lowest of all cancer funding.

- More women die of lung cancer than breast cancer.

- 15% of women with lung cancer survive; 85% of women with breast cancer survive.

- The rate of lung cancer has actually increased annually.

- The survival rate for lung cancer hasn't changed in 40 years. The five-year lung cancer survival rate is 16% for women and 12% for men.

- The five-year-survival rate for people diagnosed with Stage III or IV cancer is 5%; most people are not diagnosed with lung cancer until they are in these late stages.

- 50% of lung cancer patients are diagnosed after the cancer has metastasized (Stage IV).

- 15% of people with lung cancer never smoked.

- The risk of developing lung cancer is one in 13 for men and one in 16 for women.

- 40% of former smokers get lung cancer.

- There are many different kinds of lung cancer (different mutations with many different causes – many of which are not understood yet).

"Lung cancer is the single biggest killer among cancers, responsible for nearly one-fourth of all cancer deaths... The incidence of lung cancer has increased six-fold over the last 30 years... Lung cancer mortality has dramatically risen in women, particularly older women, and it is still rising... Between 1970 and 1994, lung cancer deaths among women over 55 increased by 400%, more than the rise in the rates of breast and colon cancer combined." from <u>The Emperor of All Maladies: A Biography of Cancer,</u> by Dr. Siddhartha Mukherjee.

And here is a poignant comment from the blog, "A Flying Elephant" by Teri Simon, another lung cancer survivor (sadly, no longer with us):

*"My goal is to inspire everyone to help end the stigma of the lung cancer patient! We simply have **got** to take smoking out of the equation! Smoking is bad for you for myriad reasons, but it is **not** the only reason why people get lung cancer! So I ask you: speak up! Tell people you know me, tell them your stories, tell them the smoking part is irrelevant. Tell them to stop blaming the victims, even if they **were** smokers! The attitude of "you brought this on yourself" is, I think (and I don't have facts to back it up), the biggest reason why research funding is so sadly low for this dread disease, this number one cancer killer of Americans. Talk sense to people, talk facts to people. Participate in activities and donate to research if you like, but mostly help me end the stigma of the lung cancer patient."* I say *ditto* to all that!

So why aren't people out marching for lung cancer? Why isn't there more fund-raising for lung cancer research? There are many reasons, but mostly...

... the stigma/blame of lung cancer – "it's caused by smoking; therefore, if you have cancer, you brought in on yourself."

... smokers' guilt and self-blame: they feel they are getting what they deserve so they don't speak up.

... not knowing that non-smokers get lung cancer.

... so many people die of lung cancer there's no one out there available to march!

What can you do to help?

- Tell everyone what you now know about these lung cancer facts; educate people so that there is more awareness and support.

- Start marching to raise funds for lung cancer research; join "Free to Breathe" events.

- Donate for lung cancer research; go to www.lungcancerpartnership.org.

And how can you prevent yourself (or your loved ones) from getting lung cancer?

- The obvious – don't smoke and don't be around smokers.

- Check for radon or asbestos exposure in your home and business.

- Get a recent chest x-ray (or, better yet, a CT scan).

- Live as stress-free as possible.

- Eat a plant-based diet and avoid dairy (for this rationale, watch the DVDs "Forks over Knives" or

"Food Matters"; read "The China Study"; and see "You Are What You Eat" and "What I've Learned About Healthy Nutrition".

- Read "Healing Myself" for other ideas on prevention.

- Keep reading my book – there's a lot of helpful information within.

I hope you will embrace our goal of stopping this epidemic of lung cancer. Your goal should be the same so that you will avoid getting lung cancer yourself. My posts are meant to help you learn all the ways to prevent lung cancer from occurring in your body. Be proactive; help yourself and help others. Let's stop all these unnecessary lung cancer deaths!

Potential Speech to a Community Group

It's likely that I won't live long enough to see my grandchildren graduate from college, or maybe even high school! I probably won't be at their weddings or other significant life events. My life is going to be cut short by lung cancer.

I am an unlikely lung cancer victim. I was never a smoker; I lived what I thought was a healthy lifestyle; I'm relatively young. How could I get cancer? The known causes of lung cancer are smoking, radon, and asbestos; I was exposed to none of these. I actually believe diet was and is a major factor, but western medicine does not recognize this factor. Doctors still don't study diet and nutrition as a preventive or healing approach to medicine, yet there are many studies that prove the links between a poor diet (dairy, processed foods, sugar, animal protein) and cancer.

In a routine chest x-ray in preparation for a lumpectomy, they found the lung cancer in my body. After surgery (removing the top lobe of my right lung and a piece of the lower lobe), chemotherapy, and radiation, the lung cancer returned into both lungs, along with a small metastasis to my brain. I was upgraded to Stage IV, which has a dire prognosis (only 15% of lung cancer patients live beyond five years; actually only 5% of late stage lung cancer patients live that long).

However, I am defying statistics as I approach the fifth year of treatment. I attribute my survival to Tarceva®, the "magic bullet" chemotherapy pill they put me on after SRS (Stereotactic RadioSurgery) to my brain. I have been tumor-free since taking the pill. It was research that found this amazing medication.

Research has actually found that lung cancer is really not one cancer; it is many different kinds of cancer with different types of mutations. So far they have found about 23 mutations, EGFR being one of the most common (which is the one I have); ALK is another common one. The value of knowing about mutations is that medications can be found to target that specific mutation. Tarceva® is known to significantly affect EGFR; ALK needs a different medication (Crizotinib). Unfortunately these medications are not permanently successful; the cancer finds a way around it eventually.

My time on Tarceva® might be almost up. The average length of time it is effective is two years; I've been taking it for over three years. I can only hope that researchers are finding another drug that I can use. The problem with lung cancer research is that it is the least funded, even though lung cancer kills more people (men and women) than breast, prostate, and colon cancer combined!

US Cancer Deaths vs. Federal Research Funding per Death

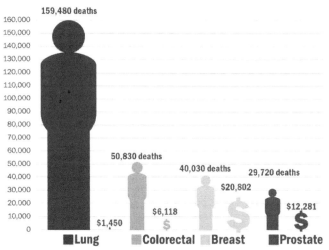

Figure ©2013 National Lung Cancer Partnership. All rights reserved.

Why is lung cancer the least funded of all cancers? Is it due to the belief that lung cancer is caused by smoking; therefore, smokers deserve what they get? (Do they really? Does anyone deserve cancer?) Or is it because they believe they know the cause (smoking), therefore no more research needs to be done? Is it because they are unaware of all the lung cancer victims who never smoked? This is *wrong*! We need to face the reality of the lung cancer epidemic and do something to stop it!

I'm here to educate you about the problem of lung cancer, ways to prevent it, and to ask your help in funding lung cancer research.

Please tell everyone you know what you have learned and visit www.lungcancerpartnership.org to donate.

Summits and Conferences

The Lung Cancer Advocacy Summit

I just returned from Nashville, Tennessee, where I attended the *5th Annual Lung Cancer Advocacy Summit* put on by the *National Lung Cancer Partnership.* The Partnership generously pays all expenses for those attending so that we will go back to our communities to advocate for lung cancer research.

There were 70 participants: 24 cancer survivors and 36 survivors of a lost loved one. People came from 28 different states. The networking was invaluable, and the sharing of personal stories was very moving. It felt comforting to know I am not alone.

We attended workshops from morning into the evening. Workshop topics included learning the facts about lung cancer, preventing and screening for lung cancer, addressing the stigma of lung cancer, creating our message and using social media to get our message out, and, mostly, exploring all the ways to advocate for lung cancer research, including legislative advocacy, consumer advocacy, community education, using the media, and fundraising.

We also visited Vanderbilt University to learn about the lung cancer research they do, as well as to witness their research in action. All very interesting and informative.

In the end we created personal action plans on how we each plan to advocate for lung cancer in our respective communities. Many people chose to organize walks/runs called "Free to Breathe," which have been very successful. (Check out www.freetobreathe.com to find a walk near your city; there are many of them scheduled across the country.) Other creative fundraising events were discussed (for example, wine walks, yogathons, danceathons, etc.). We were encouraged to participate in local Health Fairs where we can educate more people about lung cancer. Some of us will be contacting our elected officials and finding ways to get involved in legislative initiatives at the federal and local levels. Others will be writing to the media to get better coverage of lung cancer. I plan to find opportunities to speak to local community/business/school groups (and to continue to advocate for lung cancer in my blog). We all will be leaving printed materials in doctors' offices and waiting rooms, on bulletin boards, in stores and shops, etc.

The Lung Cancer Partnership will support us in every way we need by providing handouts and posters for health fairs, fact sheets, materials for other venues, an individualized power point presentation for public speaking, sample letters to the editor, and press releases. The Partnership will be available to answer any questions we may have at any time.

The goal of all of this advocacy is to get more funding for lung cancer research. I don't think I would be alive today without the research that discovered Tarceva® and its effectiveness against the EGFR mutation. At some point the cancer will become resistant to Tarceva®, but research will find a new drug to help me fight it. But without better funding there will be no research!

Research has been very effective in finding cures for breast cancer and HIV/Aids. The many voices from those survivors are what made the difference. HIV has become a chronic disease; 85% of breast cancer patients survive now (while only 15% of lung cancer patients survive). We need more voices advocating for lung cancer research; I hope you will be one of them! And please help out by telling everyone you know what you have learned and by donating what you can to save a life.

Living With Cancer - Navigating the Cancer Journey

That was the title of a free cancer conference I attended at Mass General Hospital (MGH). Over 100 patients (and friends) attended, along with a large support staff of nurses, doctors, and clinicians. Like last year's conference, I learned a lot about recent cancer research, but, more importantly, I came away with renewed hope and optimism while living with my cancer.

The first speaker, Dr. Birrer, a researcher from MGH, explained all about clinical trials, what they are, their purpose and goals, the different stages, and how they're effective. Often, being in a clinical trial saves or significantly prolongs a patient's life. His presentation was also fascinating when he showed how genetic research and testing are done. I was thrilled when he told us that there is much more hope now for living longer lives managing our cancers since there is more and more research being done and development time is much shorter.

The second speaker was the one I most resonated with: a 55-year-old woman who is a long-term lung cancer survivor. She was diagnosed in 2003 (eight years ago!) with Stage IV non-small cell lung cancer (like me, a non-smoker but, unlike me, she was EGFR negative). Doctors were able to identify the genetic mutation she has (ALK) and found the right drug (Crizotinib), which worked amazingly well; it practically eliminated her tumors! Unfortunately, a different gene has just mutated (which is very likely to happen to me), so they are now determining what other drug to use. However, the doctors are optimistic that the next drug will also be effective. She really inspired me because she is clearly living a full life while dealing with the same serious lung cancer that I have.

Another interesting presentation was a panel of five cancer survivors, each describing his or her story and current condition. Their stories were all very moving and inspiring. Later a panel of specialized MGH staff addressed emotional issues, medical concerns, nutrition, and exercise, and described the MGH programs and services available. All of this was very informative and helpful.

They gave us a free lunch so we could mix and mingle with other patients. I was thrilled to meet another breast cancer survivor who is also a life coach. We will stay in touch as we continue along our cancer journeys, focusing more on enjoying each day while trusting that we have a long life ahead of us.

Here are some interesting statistics regarding cancer survivors:

- In 1971 there were 3 million
- In 1990 there were 10 million
- In 2007 there were 12 million
- In 2020 there will be 20 million

Cancer is becoming a chronic disease, a disease of aging; we will see more and more people with cancer live longer lives.

There was a lot of talk among the participants about "chemo-brain", which is very much a side effect of chemotherapy (and radiation and medications) that affects people in a variety of ways, some more severely than others. I know I have been affected; sometimes I scare myself at my poor memory or forgetfulness. We know that forgetfulness is part of the aging process (because all my friends complain about it), but I think I have a double whammy: aging and chemotherapy. I deal with it by trying to be more focused and conscious, paying more attention to what I say and do. I write things down; I do things to force myself to use my memory (like playing Bridge), or I do things that make me use my brain (like playing Sudoku® or Scrabble®). I also ask my friends and family to be patient with me (see "Chemo Brain").

Another point addressed at the conference was what all survivors live with: fear of recurrence of their cancer or of the appearance of a different cancer (which is very common, sad to say). Many patients at the conference had multiple cancers. Unfortunately, the cancer treatments, like cat scans and radiation, can trigger new cancers. In addition to cancer, depression and anxiety are common.

Also addressed was the need to learn to deal with (and accept) the "new normal" life, including:

- cognitive impairment (chemo brain)

- poor body image (losing hair/change in hair texture and color, gaining/losing weight, losing teeth, eyesight, hearing, body rash, etc.)

- loss of dignity (for example, uncontrollable bowel problems)

- loss of work (fostering financial concerns as well as loss of identity and purpose)

Hearing my concerns voiced by so many patients and physicians was helpful; I know I'm not alone. At the same time there were lots of inspiring, encouraging, hopeful stories, and that is what I walked away with. I feel I now have a bigger support network I can draw upon whenever I need it, and I am so glad to be part of one of the best hospitals in the world!

Living Well With Cancer

I just spent the weekend at Omega Institute in Rhineback, New York, attending an excellent conference for cancer survivors.

There were over 100 participants and 10 inspiring and interesting speakers. The participants were mostly cancer survivors, mainly women with breast cancer. There were only a few of us with lung cancer, which wasn't surprising. The attendance corroborated statistics: 85% of breast cancer patients survive; 15% of lung cancer patients survive.

The speakers were from a variety of disciplines:

- Dr. Siddhartha Mukherjee, author of <u>The Emperor of All Maladies: A Biography of Cancer</u>

- Gabrielle Roth, a noted dancer and lung cancer survivor

- Lura Shopteau, psychologist and yoga teacher

- Paul Epstein, ND, a naturopathic physician and Buddhist meditation teacher

- Ruth Backman, a cancer amputee and inspirational speaker

- Skip Backus, CEO at Omega and a cancer survivor healed by "John of God"

- Kris Carr, author of <u>Crazy, Sexy Cancer</u> and <u>Crazy, Sexy Diet</u>

- Carla Goldstein, breast cancer survivor, lawyer, Omega faculty, and our MC

- a Qigong master from Sloan-Kettering Cancer Center

- Dr. Brent Bauer, Director of Complementary Medicine, Mayo Clinic

We listened to their informative and inspiring words, we practiced yoga and meditation and Qigong, we wrote in journals, we shared our stories, and we enjoyed the beauty of the lovely and relaxing environment at Omega. I also treated myself to a deep tissue massage and an hour of reflexology – divine!

I left feeling more hopeful and inspired and informed, as well as more connected to the "tribe" of growing cancer survivors. I was also convinced to incorporate more "complementary medicine" into my healing – yoga, acupuncture, massage, meditation, Qigong, to continue to eat a plant-based, sugar-free diet, and to keep on dancing!

Some of the words of wisdom from the speakers include:

- Don't be attached to the outcome of your cancer journey; be attached only to the present moment.
- One person's story will not be my cancer story.
- Cancer is my teacher.
- Your kitchen is your pharmacy; food is medicine. You are what you eat.
- Become the CEO of your health.
- Self-healing is key. Take responsibility for your own health care.
- From fierce grace and courage comes the healing.
- We need to transform loss into opportunity for growth; there is a silver lining to living with cancer.
- Grieving is a process of discovery; it's a spiritual path.
- Change is inevitable; transformation is intentional.
- Cancer transforms us, often for the better.
- Healing is a soup and the key ingredient is me.

- Focus on healing rather than on curing; there is a healing path.

How do we get cancer? *Some words of wisdom from the speakers:*

Dr. Mukherjee states that cancer is an age-related disease. As we get older our immune system becomes weaker so that it can't fight the cancer cells that mutate daily in our body. He did say that researchers have learned that cancer is weak, but they still haven't figured out all the ways to find the weak points. The good news is that the mortality rate is going down for many cancers; each year there are more and more cancer survivors (sadly, not for lung cancer... yet!).

Kris Carr focused on diet, emphasizing that we need a predominantly alkaline diet; most of our diets are highly acidic. Animal protein, filled with anti-nutrients, is highly acidic, has no anti-oxidants, no phytonutrients, and no fiber, which are all essential ingredients for a healthy diet. Studies prove that casein, found in 87% of dairy, causes tumors. Milk also contains the 1GF1 growth factor, a hormone meant to help a 70 lb. calf grow to 1,000 lbs. in six months. Calves get weaned; people don't!

Kris insists that we need to eat a plant-based diet (also avoid sugar and processed foods) if we want to prevent or to heal cancer. She also pointed out that we do not need to worry about getting enough protein (which seems to be most people's concern). A 130 lb. woman needs only 40 grams of protein daily, yet each day the average person ingests 100-120 grams of protein! Kris walks her talk: as a 12 year, Stage IV cancer survivor, she lives a healthy, vibrant life. I found her to be incredibly inspiring and informative, a beautiful person and a motivational speaker. I highly suggest you read her diet book and check out her website: www.crazysexylife.com.

Dr. Bauer presented a PowerPoint presentation showing the research recently done at the Mayo Clinic proving the positive effects of using complementary medicine modalities to reduce stress related to cancer.

Gabrielle Roth, creator of "The Effects of 5 Rhythms Movement Therapy on Cancer Survivors", showed us how dancing can help us with our healing (see "Keep On Dancing").

Cancer Conversations on Cancer's Changing Landscape

Last night I attended a panel presentation put on by the cancer centers of Beverly and Addison Gilbert Hospitals and Beth Israel Deaconess Medical Center. The panelists were doctors of various specialties (breast cancer, lung cancer, prostate cancer, colorectal cancer, leukemia/lymphoma) who spoke about the latest research in their area. Their presentations were informative, although I had already heard much of the information. Some concepts that were new to me were:

- SRS (Stereotactic RadioSurgery - which I had) is now used effectively for early stage lung cancer tumors.

- Radiation may cause more harm than necessary (for example, cause other cancers); therefore, doctors are cutting back on giving it, especially after breast lumpectomies.

- "Wait and see" is becoming more of a standard of treatment for men with prostate cancer; quality of life is becoming more of a focus.

- Palliative care is now used for people in active treatment as well as for end-stage care.

- Drug shortages – unavailability – are not of serious concern… yet.

- There is a need to focus more on cancer survivorship and ways to manage chronic cancer.

- There still is no effective screening strategy (like mammograms or colonoscopies) for lung cancer; cat scans do not seem to provide proper preventive screening.

- (note: a more recent report seems to indicate that cat scans are effective in screening for lung cancer in earlier stages).

- The oral chemo pill, Erlotinib (Tarceva®), is often a superior treatment modality than infusion chemotherapy for patients testing positive for the EGFR mutation.

- There are actually 54 different types of lung cancer; it's all about mutations now.

When I asked about Tarceva® and what happens when it stops working, I wasn't happy, but not surprised, with the answer. The lung specialist confirmed that cancer tumors are smart. Cancer adapts, becomes resistant, and finds ways to bypass the medication by eventually creating novel mutations. So, I know my time is limited on this drug. I just hope I'm one of the few people who manage to stay on it for five to seven years, not just the two year average. And, once Tarceva® becomes ineffective, I can hope that by then there will be a new drug that will be effective.

I asked the panelists what recommendations they had for prevention strategies, especially for healthy nutrition. I was very disappointed, but not surprised, at the response to this question. First they mentioned medications that are being used for prevention, all a drug-based approach. There was no mention of the recent studies that show that complementary therapies like yoga, acupuncture, meditation, etc. are quite effective in reducing stress (which is linked to cancer), nor of the many studies that show the correlations between cancer and dairy or animal-protein. The only comment from the panel regarding nutrition was about supplements and how there is no proof that supplements help anyone be more healthy (I agree).

Doctors need to be more educated on the alternative ways to prevent and manage cancer... ways that are proven to be successful, such as eating a plant-based diet. The cynics say doctors and hospitals are not motivated to recommend nutritional therapy due to financial considerations; cancer is big business! Even if a doctor "means well" there is probably an "incentive-caused bias" to continue to use traditional cancer treatments. There is also the lack of nutrition education in most medical schools, so most doctors are unaware of the preventive and healing nature of proper nutrition. I believe doctors want to help cure their patients and will access all types of information to do that, it's just that there is so much information out there that it's hard for them to keep up. This is another reason we need to become our own health care advocate!

I did feel more optimistic at the end of the panel presentation. They concluded by saying we might not be curing cancer, but we are learning to control it, thus more and more cancer patients will live for many years with cancer as a chronic disease. I plan to be one of them!

Medication & Treatment

Managing Medication Side Effects

I have had to deal with over 23 different side effects from Tarceva®, the chemotherapy pill I have been taking for over three years. I had a couple of new side effects recently: paronychia (in-grown toe nails) and blepharitis ("dandruff" of the eye). Most of the side effects are related to the extreme dehydration the pill causes – dry eyes, dry hair, dry skin, dry nostrils, dry mouth, etc. There are other side effects, including the most annoying – rash and diarrhea – but I won't bore you with the entire list.

I try to look at the bright side of all this: side effects mean the pill is working! (I also seem to be gaining a new vocabulary and knowledge of other medical conditions!)

I know sometimes they say that the treatment is worse than the disease. Some cancer patients choose to stop their chemotherapy treatment when their side effects become too unbearable, and many people say they would never go through chemotherapy if recommended for them.

A recent article in the AARP bulletin mentions that millions of people each day suffer from the side effects of their medications, then they have to take drugs to treat the side effects of those drugs. According to Dr. Gordon Schiff of Harvard Medical School, *"…maybe the initial drug is essential… but when you're taking a drug to treat the side effect of a drug that is treating the side effect of another drug, it gets to be rather a house of cards."*

It's hard to know how much or how long to tolerate treatment, especially if you're uncertain about whether the side effects will create an even worse condition, or whether the medication will actually be effective. While there is a basic understanding about the effectiveness and effects of medication, each person's biochemistry is different. And many cancer medications are new, especially those in clinical trials, and the expected outcomes are often undetermined and unpredictable.

I'm lucky, I guess, because it's obvious the medication I'm taking (Tarceva®) is very effective: no tumors seen in my lungs for over three years! However, I have another friend whose medications continue to cause varying degrees of discomfort and it's unclear whether they're working or not, so she gets discouraged.

Before I was taking oral chemotherapy, I had traditional chemotherapy infusions. Each all-day infusion (four of them with three weeks in between each session) caused incrementally painful side effects: hair loss, nausea, mouth sores, fatigue, and more. I couldn't have handled them for much longer than I did and I don't think I would choose to go through that again if prescribed! I understand why people stop their treatments if they have to deal with side effects like that for long term.

Also, when you're taking a drug, it's not always easy to tell whether a side effect is related to the drug, to the underlying medical condition, or to a different health problem entirely. It can all be very confusing and discouraging and uncomfortable… and often painful.

However, when the drug(s) work, it's a miracle. Mine is a miracle. I'm living a full and meaningful and happy life thanks to Tarceva® (and my new healthy diet, I'm sure), so I can put up with all the annoying side effects it creates. It's worth it, don't you think?

Chemo Brain

"Chemo Brain" is a reality. When I first heard people talk about it, I dismissed it as a joke. But it's no joke.

I scare myself sometimes with my forgetfulness, but then I remind myself that (#1) I'm old – 67 – and (#2) I've had a lot of chemotherapy drugs coursing through my body for years, and (#3) I'm still taking a daily chemo pill.

All my older friends complain of forgetfulness; it is certainly a phenomenon of the aging process. Brain cells die out and there are too many brain cells to access the information we need right away (often we remember later - phew!). I expect to have a certain amount of forgetfulness due to my age, but I think my memory lapses go way beyond the norm because of chemo. It's frustrating, it's embarrassing, and it's scary.

Just last night I misplaced my car keys after having dinner with my son in Boston. I needed to drive home to Gloucester (an hour away). The waiters, maître d', customers, and I searched all over: at the table where we ate, in the restroom, in the lobby, outside – the keys were nowhere! I started to panic; how would I get home?

I live alone, so there was no one to help out. Finally, I found the keys on a park bench near where we had walked en route to the car. I have no idea why I left them there and I had no recollection of putting them down. Scary!

There have been many other incidences of this type of forgetfulness and mindlessness, but I can't remember them at the moment!

I also notice I say words that I don't mean. For instance, today I told a friend I was sitting in front of the "Great Barrier Reef" when I meant "Good Harbor Beach."

The other day I told friends I'm reading War and Peace when actually I'm reading Anna Karenina.

I've heard other cancer patients who have had chemotherapy complain of "chemo brain." There are a number of blogs written by cancer survivors who comment on the difficulty of dealing with it. At the MGH cancer conference this year, a speaker on a panel totally blanked out on what she was saying; she blamed it on her "chemo brain."

I guess it's just another thing I have to learn to live with in my "new normal" life. I just hope that my friends and family will continue to be understanding and supportive (they are, of course). And I also need to forgive myself when it happens.

I am doing my best to learn new strategies to be more mindful. I'm playing Bridge and Scrabble® and Sudoku®; I'm meditating and doing yoga; I'm focusing on the present. I just hope I don't forget to put all these strategies into practice!

It's Not About the Hair...

...that's what I tell myself at least. But now my hair is not *my* hair, it's some alien outcropping that I am having a hard time liking (and numerous hair dressers are having a hard time styling). My friends say it looks "interesting" and "different" and "unique." I know they are being kind. I think it looks "unattractive" and "unappealing" and just plain "boring."

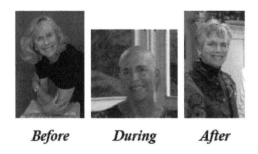

Before   *During*   *After*

Losing my hair to chemotherapy three years ago was a shock, but expected. I didn't mind being bald as much as I thought I would. I had fun wearing different types of wigs and scarves, and even the bald look was quite attractive, I was told. At least when one is bald, people know why; there's a certain amount of sympathy and understanding. (And there are many compatriots in the "bald club.") My hair grew back in unrecognizable curls, but eventually my natural straight blonde (and some gray) hair emerged. For the first time, I had short hair and it did look kind of cute (everyone said).

But lately my hair has been turning curly again – even frizzy; it feels like a Brillo® pad. The reason for this hair change is Tarceva®. The chemicals in the pill are causing permanent chemo-hair! Of course I need to stop whining and be glad that the pill has been keeping the tumors away all this time. And I am glad! I prefer no tumors with frizzy hair to tumors with beautiful hair. We all hope I can tolerate being on this pill for many more years, so I just have to get used to my new look.

Losing one's hair is a humbling experience. It is a loss of identity; it's a loss of one's image of oneself. I often thought my hair was my best feature. But when I think of all the women who have had to deal with the loss of their breasts, I realize that my hair loss is nothing compared to dealing with their losses.

I tell myself I need an "attitude adjustment" (see "It's All About Attitude") and create an "attitude of gratitude" that I'm still here today, feeling healthy and happy, surrounded by friends and family who care about me and not about how my hair looks.

It's really not about the hair!

Tarceva® Trials and Tribulations

Tarceva® (generic name: Erlotinib) is a "tyrosine kinase inhibitor used to treat certain types of advanced metastatic lung cancer." It's a miracle chemotherapy drug for those of us with the EGFR (Epidermal Growth Factor Receptor) mutation. When the EGFR is mutated, it is stuck in the "on" position, meaning the cancerous cells keep reproducing. Tarceva® stops the cancerous cell membrane from telling the cell nucleus to reproduce, thus, for a small proportion of lung cancer patients, cancer growth can be arrested for months, even years. Instead of *carpet-bombing* all the cells – cancerous and non-cancerous alike (which is what most chemotherapy does) – Tarceva® targets certain genetic aspects of *only* the cancer cells. I seem to be one of that small proportion whose cancer growth is arrested! I have been tumor-free since I started taking Tarceva® in 2010.

However, dealing with the side effects from this pill has been incredibly challenging.

There is a long list of possible side effects listed in the drug information sheet: acne, diarrhea, dry skin, fatigue, hair loss or excessive hair growth, headache, loss of appetite, stomach pain, mouth sores or ulcers, nausea, upset stomach, vomiting, weight loss; and severe eye dryness, irritation, redness, along with vision problems. Most of these side effects I have already experienced. Hopefully, the others will not develop!

First there was a very uncomfortable and unattractive rash all over my face and chest. I had the acne I never had as a teenager; whiteheads and red bumps were everywhere. My chest itched unbearably. The other major side effect was diarrhea, unpredictable and uncontrollable, with painful cramps. Fortunately this symptom has gotten more controllable over time, and the rash seems to be mostly gone. The body adjusts.

Unfortunately, other side effects developed. The worst of these to manage has been my eye problems; dry eyes have become a major pain. My eyes are always itching and burning and red. In the morning I can't even open them without first putting in eye drops. I worry that my eyesight is being affected, but so far eye tests don't show any deterioration. Eye plugs, inserted into the tear ducts, have helped a lot, as does frequent use of eye drops. This is *the most* challenging of all the side effects. I have another, even more serious eye problem: eyelashes growing *inward*. I had to go to the emergency room two times because the pain was so unbearable. The eyelash scratched my cornea every time I blinked. I saw five different ophthalmologists before the aberrant eyelash was found! (It's a rare condition). Now I have to be vigilant as another lash is sure to grow inward at some point. It seems contradictory, but my eyelashes also grow *outwardly* much longer and more erratically.

My hair seems to be affected in many different ways. Eyebrows, facial, and nose hair appear to be growing more abundantly. At the same time the hair on my arms and legs doesn't grow much at all, nor does the hair on my head. In fact it seems I am developing a receding hairline. Fortunately I have always had very thick hair.

Dry mouth is another annoying side effect; I have very little saliva. I'm sure this is affecting my taste buds, as things do not taste the same. Food flavors seem to be muted, wine tastes acidic, and I can't tolerate spicy food. Dry hair (see "It's Not About the Hair...") has been a challenge to style; dry skin is causing premature wrinkles. Every part of my body is dry, dry, dry!

Nausea also seems to be a constant companion. I frequently have an upset stomach before or after I eat; I even vomit once in awhile. I don't seem to have much of an appetite, and I have lost a lot of weight.

I have a good side effect: I'm not fatigued; I always seem to have a lot of energy. I am glad for this!

Cracked fingers, split fingernails, in-grown toenails (paronychias) have also been constant companions.

Another challenging side effect is extreme sun sensitivity. I get a bad sun rash on my chest and arms as well as a *very swollen* and *very painful* lip whenever I'm in the sun. Last summer my doctor ordered me out of the sun completely for two weeks because of my swollen lip; this summer I ended up in the emergency room (see "Not So Lazy Days!"). Because my lip was red and raw from the sun, it had developed a nasty bacterial infection. So I must be very careful when I'm in the sun. I wear a broad-brim hat or I cover my lip with a facemask.

Lately I've developed a side effect that scares me a little: my right lung really hurts when I sneeze or cough or even take a deep breath. I suspect this is a result of my lung surgery scar tissue, not Tarceva®. I certainly hope it is not a symptom of growing tumors. (*Update:* A recent bone scan showed "all clear." The pain is diagnosed as *costochondritis*, an inflammation of the junctions between cartilage and ribs, a common condition of unknown cause that is not related to cancer, which goes away without treatment).

I yawn a lot (and not because I'm tired). I also notice that I have trouble catching my breath whenever I over-exert (hike, bike, dance), but that could be because I'm just not in good enough aerobic shape. I need to work out more often.

I've now counted over 25 different side effects that I've experienced (and am experiencing) since I started taking Tarceva®, including chemo brain (see "Chemo Brain"). Another lung cancer blogger who is on Tarceva® mentioned that he has had over 80 side effects since being on the drug (for over four years). Tarceva® is a difficult drug to manage; many cancer patients can't even tolerate it. It is such an important drug, there is a whole blog ("Tarceva® Divas and Dudes") devoted to it – www.inspired.com/lungcancer – where patients share stories, answer questions, and provide support. I have found the site very helpful. The patients writing on the blog often know more than the doctors. They have even created a long list of "Tarceva® side effect busters."

All my side effects from Tarceva® make it hard to ignore that I have lung cancer, which is a bummer. However, I have learned to manage quite well, and feel that I live just fine with little interference in my day-to-day, "new normal" life. I just need to be sure there is always a toilet nearby and a local emergency room! It's fairly certain that I will develop more side effects as long as I am on this chemo pill, but I always remind myself that these side effects mean the pill is working. I also have to be aware that some conditions I develop (like *costochondritis*) may not have anything to do with Tarceva® or cancer.

Without Tarceva® I don't think I'd be alive today, so I'm very happy to be on this miracle drug! I actually hope to live with these side effects for many more years to come.

Dancing Through Cancer

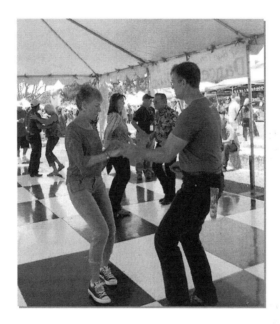

Zydeco Dancing

How Can I Be Dancing Through Cancer?

Attitude is everything and dancing helps my attitude! My friends always comment on my positive, hopeful attitude throughout all my cancer treatments and management. But I tell them my attitude is one of the things I have control over. I choose to focus on the positive because I know it will help me have a better quality of life. I can't control the rogue cancer cells, but I can choose how I react to what is going on. I can choose how I spend my time, with whom I spend my time, what I eat, what I do for exercise, and how I play. I know all of these factors affect how I manage my cancer (see "Healing Myself"). Dancing, especially, affects my mood positively and joyfully, so it seems an appropriate metaphor for managing to live with cancer.

So I dance (Zydeco) as often as I can!! When I dance I forget my condition; I feel healthy and confident and attractive and playful and energized. I have fun with my dance partners; I sometimes have *peak experiences*. I love the way the music infuses me with positive vibrations. Dancing helps me focus on the joyful aspects of my life; it helps me be in the present moment and be totally *in the flow*. I tell my friends that having a positive attitude may be easier for me because I feel good most of the time. I feel like dancing! I usually have a lot of energy and my side effects are manageable. Thus I can ignore my disease and focus on enjoying my life, especially when I dance! I am choosing to live life to the fullest each and every day. You can make this choice too. I hope I inspire you!

Keep On Dancing

Gabrielle Roth, a lung cancer survivor and professional dancer, presented a program at the "Living Well with Cancer" conference I recently attended. She got us all up and dancing in order to experience the power of dancing through cancer.

Roth is the creator of a program: "The Effects of 5 Rhythms Movement Therapy on Cancer Survivors." The results of the studies for this program showed significant reductions of stress, depression, anxiety, and intolerance of uncertainty, and increases in quality of life, positive body image, and serenity.

Why else dance? Dancing helps us get in touch with our bodies, and thus feel our emotions. Dancing activates adrenalin and other positive hormones. It's impossible to feel fear or be stressed when one feels joyful. Dancing is a joyful expression, even a peak experience, but mostly dancing is just plain *fun*!

A recent study in the *New England Journal of Medicine* showed that *"recreational activities positively affected the minds of older people, and the number one activity cited was dancing. Dancing requires memorizing steps and sequences and getting your feet and body to coordinate with what your mind is telling you. In other words, dancing integrates various brain functions at the same time, and according to the study, that helps the brain regenerate. In some cases dancing can even reduce the risk of dementia."*

Why I Love Zydeco Dancing

I go dancing as often as possible. When I dance I feel totally alive and happy and joyful; I'm living completely in the moment while I move my body in sync with my partner, infused with the music, energized, and feeling fabulous. When I dance I forget I have cancer.

I've created a list (that keeps on growing) of all the reasons I love to dance Zydeco:

1. The skill: there's always the opportunity to learn more dance steps and improve (from lessons, as well as from other dancers).

2. The challenge: of improving and of following good leaders.

3. The music: is always so moving and inspiring; there are always live bands.

4. The exercise: dancing can be very aerobic!

5. The opportunity: to learn new dance steps by being a follower; every male leader dances differently, so it's fun to follow different leads.

6. The inspiration: it's wonderful to watch the many amazing dancers on the dance floor and to learn from them and get inspired.

7. The connections: being single, there is always a possibility of meeting someone (a new friend? a new romance?).

8. The community: it's such a friendly dance community; everyone is always welcoming. I love sharing the experience with a friend and introducing Zydeco dancing to them.

9. The playfulness: dancers express their joy and happiness on the dance floor. We laugh a lot!

10. The timing: the dances start early and end early so we can get our sleep!

11. The feeling: I feel confident and beautiful and sexy and happy when I dance, and these feelings carry over off the dance floor.

12. The hormones: adrenalin and endorphins kick in!

13. At dances one can "reinvent oneself" - you can be whoever you want to be and wear whatever you want on the dance floor.

14. Dancing can be a *peak experience*: *a kind of transpersonal and ecstatic state particularly tinged with themes of euphoria, harmonization, and interconnectedness.* One can also feel a sense of being in *flow*: *a mental state in which a person performing an activity is fully immersed in a feeling of energized focus, full involvement, and enjoyment.*

15. Dancing is a type of non-verbal communication (which, they say, taps into and develops the right brain, and which helps hold off the aging process).

16. While dancing there is always male/female touching (sometimes, for single people, this is the only opposite sex touching they're getting); sometimes there's dirty dancing (with the right partner).

17. Dancing is a great equalizer: it doesn't matter what you do professionally, your race or color or age, how fat or thin you are, how tall or short you are – if you can dance, you're welcome and desirable!

18. The dances are about dancing, not about picking someone up; these are not singles dances. People dance for all the reasons listed here. People usually switch up and get a new partner after each song in order to experience the variety of dancing styles.

19. The dance festivals are full of music for days, with a variety of live bands and dancers from all over the country. There's also ethnic food, clothes and jewelry, musician workshops and jams, and dance lessons.

20. Zydeco dancing is just plain FUN!!

What Others Say About Zydeco Dancing

Here are some responses from my dance partners:

"Laurie, spoken like a true Zydeco junkie! Ditto to every one of your 20 reasons (of course, Reason 5 for me would be 'Experiencing the variety of female responses to my leading').

You've pretty much covered the territory. The only things I could add would be:

(a) An elaboration of Reason 14: Something very special happens when you can achieve perfect resonance with your partner and with the music, when everything is in sync, when you're feeling the music through your partner's body. There's (almost) no higher euphoria.

(b) The tango has been described as 'the vertical expression of a horizontal desire.' Zydeco, too, is a perfect sublimation of that horizontal desire. An artful metaphor and simulation (I tell myself) of the horizontal act. So the dance serves for me as a theatrical experience in which I'm both actor and audience. But maybe that's what you meant by your Reason 13."

"Hi Laurie, Wow, I just love all the reasons, so I had to read them over and over as I was identifying with them. I hadn't thought about it much, but as I re-read number 11, I started to realize how much more confident and happy I have become since I began Zydeco dancing. The minute I walk into a Zydeco dance, I feel tremendous joy and love, which can only be topped by the thought of my two beautiful grandsons!"

"Laurie: Dancing is an amazing thing... an exuberant experience... a kind of joyful spiritual ecstasy for me. As a leader I try to communicate with my partner through dance not so much as a leader/follower relationship, but more as equal co-partners. And I work hard to try to bring out the very best in my dance partners... what they are feeling in the music and what style they dance best. And sometimes it creates something that neither of us knew we had inside us to come out and be freed through dance. There is an intimacy when that happens that I have not found anywhere else with my shoes on! Dancing can be a 'one heart and four legs' experience when we are totally connected to the passionate music.

Dancing calls on all our senses and faculties: touch, sight, hearing, smell, and taste. It takes us to our real age (who we are) and not our chronological age (how old we are). We return to our optimum child-like state of play: safe, secure, free from worry, in the moment, sharing, loving, without care."

"It's a partner dance – a place for men and women to meet each other and to hold each other, using known steps to create together a movement poetry. Once the steps are in your body-memory, the joy begins. Moving to the music, the world disappears as you are one with the universe. It's Magic!"

"Hi Laurie, That's a pretty inclusive list of reasons you enjoy Zydeco, and I suspect most dancers would share just about all of them. It's good to see them in print because it causes one to reflect personally on each one of them. It's also important because none of us is dancing alone. It's a community of dancers engaged in couple dancing, and it is both helpful, as well as a healthy thing to consider what others are seeking in the dance experience of which we are all a contributing part if we all hope to find our maximum joy when we come together. I have a few more of my own, perhaps with some redundancy:

1. It's a friendly, open, and supportive community.
2. It's a non-competitive atmosphere – no egos, just enjoyment.
3. The dance form is very accessible.
4. The pre-dance lesson gives beginners everything they need to get started and set out with some degree of comfort.
5. The dance style is not rigid, and there is plenty of room for individual expression.
6. Many experienced dancers make it a point to dance with beginners and make them feel welcome.

7. It is satisfying to help newcomers. For some of them it will open a whole new world of joy and satisfaction, just as it did for many of us. What a wonderful gift!

8. It meets an elemental human need, largely unmet in our uptight, non-touching society, for the tactile satisfaction of friendly physical contact with others, and those of the opposite sex in particular.

9. The challenge and pleasure of the non-verbal conversation that is dance. How will our dialog proceed? What will we talk about? Will it be a wonderful give and take? Playful? Flowing? Will I find treasure? Will it be a brilliant conversation? Will we soar magically away?

10. The music is joyful and energizing.

11. The philosophy of "Laissez les bons temps rouler" ("let the good times roll") can be a healthful one to embrace – a refreshing and restorative island in a daily sea of tumult.

12. It makes one feel happy and more alive."

Overheard on the dance floor:

"I feel like a different person on the dance floor... confident and competent!"

"I could die tonight and be happy!" Response from listener: "I think I have died and I'm already in heaven!"

The Joys of Zydeco Dancing

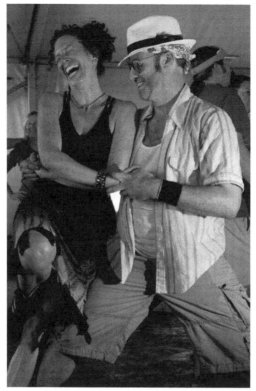

photo by Ryan Hodgson-Rigsbee • www.rhrphoto.com

To watch some great examples of zydeco dancing, go to *YouTube* and check out the following:

*Harold on Louisiana
*Zydeco Dancing (in kitchen)
*Preston Frank Grass Roots 2010
*Louisiana Zydeco Live8
*Zydeco dancing at Breaux Bridge

To check out a festival, Google "Rhythm & Roots" at Ninigret Park. To find a Zydeco dance in your area, go to www.arng.org.

Dancing Through My Life

I've always loved to dance. My earliest memories are of dancing at home with my mother and sister. My mother was a good dancer and she loved to teach us how to jitterbug, cha cha, salsa, or do the Balboa. She enrolled us in dance classes all the time: ballroom dancing, ballet, tap, even hula! I loved it all.

In junior high school I liked going to the monthly cotillion dances where we learned all types of ballroom dancing: waltz, fox trot, swing, cha cha, and polka. I was good at it. Those were the days of rock 'n roll: Buddy Holly, Richie Valens, Elvis, Chubby Checker, Jerry Lee Lewis, Ray Charles were some of my favorites. Their songs were so inspiring and fun to dance to; I still like to dance to their music (see "My 50th Class Reunion")!

When we moved to Spain when I was 14, I learned to dance Flamenco.

In high school, in Spain, we Americans would all go to the "teen club" to dance every weekend. That's where I learned to do the Twist and the Shimmy and the Pony, etc. My senior year I went on local television to demonstrate the Twist with another classmate. I was chosen "Best Dancer" of my senior class.

In college I was on the synchronized swim team; I loved it because it was like dancing to music in the water.

Music and dancing first brought my husband-to-be and me together; we shared that same passion. Over the years, our love of music kept us connected and involved. While living on a Navy Base in Puerto Rico we would give dance parties instead of boring dinner parties. Later, living in Annisquam, Massachusetts, I became Chairwoman of the Recreation Committee at the Yacht Club so that I could ensure that we had better dances. The music and DJs were carefully chosen; we really livened things up with our rock 'n roll dances.

After my divorce, I discovered Country Dancing. I would drive to a nearby dance club where I learned the "two-step" and line dances and re-learned country swing and waltz.

Then I found West Coast Swing. I preferred the music and loved the sexy dance patterns. I took many lessons and went to weekly dances, but it is a challenging dance that I never quite mastered.

I moved on to Latin Dancing: Salsa and Merengue and Bachata. In Cambridge I lived near a Salsa Club that I went to as often as possible. In Cabarete, Dominican Republic, where we owned a condo, I would dance with the locals and learned a lot of interesting dance moves. For years I sought out many opportunities for Latin dancing in the Boston area.

I even learned to Tango a bit when I lived in Argentina for two months.

But then I discovered Zydeco! I love this dance for so many reasons (see "Why I Love Zydeco Dancing"). I find as many dances as I can locally, and I go to as many festivals as I can (San Diego, Rhode Island, Connecticut). I just went to Lafayette, Louisiana, "the home of Zydeco" (see "Dancing In the New Year: 2013"). Zydeco is my dance of choice now; it's getting me through cancer joyfully.

Dancing has certainly been an important part of my life and has enriched it immensely. It has brought me friends and lovers (and a husband); it has challenged me and taught me new skills (thus expanding my brain power); it has relaxed, as well as excited me; it has provided me with many peak experiences. Dancing always gets me through my bleak moments and helps me to experience joy in life. Now, dancing is helping me manage to live with lung cancer. I hope to keep on dancing 'til I die – *Dancing Through Cancer!*

Milestones

Milestones become very important when one has lung cancer; you begin living your life hoping to achieve the next milestone ("just let me live long enough to... take this trip, or... see this event, or... go to this festival, etc."). I celebrate each milestone with satisfaction and hope... hope to reach many more milestones.

Birthdays

May 3, 2008 *- Diagnosed with Breast Cancer (DCIS) - then lung cancer!*

May 3, 2009 *- Surgery/Chemo/Radiation Failure*

May 3, 2010 *- Tarceva® Works Miracles: Tumors Gone!*

May 3, 2011 - Happy Birthday to Me!

I turned 66 this week. Three years ago (when I was shockingly diagnosed with lung cancer right around my 63rd birthday), I wasn't sure I'd see this day. But here I am! Is it a miracle? Maybe.

I count myself as one of the many (and growing number of) cancer survivors who are benefitting from the years and years of cancer research and treatment. We are the new face of cancer. Mass General Hospital (MGH) now has a Cancer Survivor Center to help cancer survivors live with their "new normal" life. There was never a need for a survivor center in the past because there were not enough cancer survivors. I plan to be as involved as I can in the Center in order to help other survivors.

I think I'm also benefitting from living a new, healthier lifestyle with better nutrition (mostly plant-based, non-dairy, limited sugar), less stress, and by using alternative, holistic therapies. I am especially grateful that I'm still here (and doing well) because the survival rate for lung cancer continues to be low. Statistics show only a 5% five-year survival rate while survival rates for other cancers have really improved (85% five-year survival rate for breast cancer). Most people are shocked by these statistics.

Research (which generates funding) makes all the difference, and it's obvious where all the funding is going. Breast cancer activists are everywhere and very visible. HIV activists changed the sure death prognosis for AIDS victims. Where are the lung cancer activists? Most are probably dead, so they aren't around to increase the public's awareness of the need for lung cancer funding for research. Each year 160,000 people die of lung cancer. Fifteen percent of newly diagnosed patients never smoked. Did you know *that lung cancer kills more people than breast, prostate, colon, pancreatic, and liver cancer combined? Yet it's the least funded!* (See **US Cancer Deaths vs. Federal Research Funding per Death** Graph in my "Potential Speech to a Community Group")

This is unacceptable! We need to help raise awareness of the need for funding and we need to have our own marches and events. I hope you'll join in this fight to kill lung cancer before it kills too many more people (see www.nationallungcancerpartnership.org).

If you have lungs, you too are at risk!

I feel more hopeful about surviving lung cancer after reading Dr. Siddhartha Mukherjee's book, The Emperor of All Maladies: A Biography of Cancer. Toward the end of the book he says, *"The mortality for nearly every major form of cancer – lung, breast, colon, and prostate – has continuously dropped for fifteen straight years... Mortality has declined by 1% every year... This is... an unprecedented decline in the history of the disease. Cancer is losing its power..."* Yea!

We still don't know the causes of most cancers; scientists cannot explain how cancers continue to proliferate endlessly. Identifying genomes, finding and targeting cancer mutations, seems to be the focus of research right now, but more research needs to be done and we need money for that. Every patient's cancer is unique because every cancer genome is unique. Once a mutation is identified the "right" drug can be used for treatment. That's why I'm lucky, apparently, that they have identified the mutated gene I have (EGFR), because Tarceva®, the pill I take daily, is very effective; it is keeping away my tumors (for now). I trust that once my pill stops working there will be a new one that will be just as effective.

To keep pace with this malady – cancer – we need to keep inventing and reinventing, learning and unlearning strategies. I know that's what's happening, and I'm hopeful. And I'm very happy to celebrate another birthday, trusting that I'll have many more to come!!

May 3, 2012 - Another Happy Birthday

I celebrated another birthday! Four years ago I was diagnosed with breast cancer, then lung cancer… not exactly the happy birthday gifts I wanted! At the time, my doctor told me that two more birthdays might be all I'd celebrate. But, here I am, celebrating my sixty-seventh birthday, post-cancer diagnosis. I feel great, and I'm optimistic that I will be celebrating many more to come. I'm determined to change the morbid statistical landscape of cancer.

Birthdays are wonderful. We can be "queens for the day." Family and friends, even acquaintances, take the time to wish us happiness. I received so many calls, emails, Facbook posts, cards, flowers, and gifts wishing me well. I felt so special and loved. I am so very grateful for all the rich and loving relationships in my life. Words are inadequate to express my sincere appreciation for all they give me.

Birthdays are also a time when we treat ourselves, and I certainly did: I had a massage, got my hair done, took a yoga class, went out to dinner with friends, and even bought myself a little gift. Birthdays are days we give ourselves permission to indulge and enjoy; I know how to do that quite well!

Why wait for birthdays to treat ourselves? Why wait for birthdays to tell the people we care about that we love them? When was the last time you told someone how much he or she means to you, or did something nice for him or her, or gave him or her something they wanted for no reason?

Let's use birthdays to remind ourselves that we can celebrate each and every day. We can treat ourselves every day; we can treat our friends and family every day. I certainly am celebrating that I'm still alive and well and I'm celebrating all the rich relationships in my life. A very happy birthday indeed!

May 3, 2013 - Five Year Anniversary of Lung Cancer Survival

As I approach my 68th birthday and the five-year anniversary of my lung cancer diagnosis, I feel great. I am surrounded by friends and family who love and support me every day; I live in a beautiful place on the water; I have lots of energy and am able to do just about anything I want: I travel, I sail and kayak and bike and hike and swim; I walk the beach; I meditate and practice yoga; I dance as often as I can. My life is richer than it has ever been; I'm happier than I have ever been. I appreciate each and every day, and am optimistic that I will be celebrating many more birthdays to come.

Planning For the New Year: 2012

It must be a good sign that I am planning for the New Year. I guess I expect to be around for a lot longer, continuing to enjoy a rich and fulfilling life.

- I plan to continue to spend as much quality time as I can with my family and friends.

- I plan to keep on traveling: Costa Rica and California to visit family, and now planning a trip to Southeast Asia!

- Since it looks like I am going to live longer than expected, I plan to rev up my work schedule and start offering coaching to other cancer survivors (see "Offering Cancer Coaching").

- I plan to continue to work as a consultant for Right Management, Teacher Education Institute, and Outward Bound Professionals.

- I plan to keep on dancing, sailing, kayaking, swimming, hiking, biking, skiing, practicing yoga, etc.

- I even find myself planning, along with my special girlfriends, to live together in a women's community of caring and support in about ten years. I am optimistic!

I continue to feel great, so it's easy to forget that I have Stage IV lung cancer!

I always seem to have a lot of energy and I've learned to manage (and mostly ignore) the multitude of side effects from my chemo-pill, Tarceva® (see "Tarceva® Trials and Tribulations"). I'm sure that eating well – mostly a plant-based diet minimizing sugar and dairy – contributes to my positive energy and well-being. Maintaining an attitude of optimism and hope is certainly helping. It's a "new ball game" now regarding (lung) cancer treatment and care, so I am optimistic that new drugs and treatment options will be available to me as the years go on. I plan to be one of the many long-term survivors. 2011 was a good year: tumor free after each cat scan/MRI/mammogram.

I did my best to "live each day as if it were my last." Receiving a cancer diagnosis has a way of focusing our attention on what is most important in life and helping us appreciate every day and each relationship. This is what I focus on:

- Less work and more play.

- Spending more quality time with friends (especially my women's group) and family (especially my three grandchildren, my two sons, my niece, my cousin, my mother).

- Traveling to Costa Rica, France and Spain, California, New York, Cape Cod, Australia and New Zealand, Southeast Asia... and beyond.

- Sailing, kayaking, biking, hiking, skiing, walking...

- Dancing Zydeco a lot.

- Healthy living: eating well, exercising, practicing yoga, and getting massages... (see "Healing Myself").

- Continuing to educate myself about ways to live well with cancer.

- Writing in my blog (and publishing this book) in order to share my journey with you.

Sadly, this year wasn't all good: I lost three special friends to cancer (and a stroke); I will always cherish, and never forget, each of them. Their abrupt deaths continue to remind me to live mindfully and gratefully each and every day. A recent article describing a study of women who survive cancer really resonated with me.

Women who survive cancer….

- Face down death and live each day as if it were their last.

- Give up "being beautiful" and focus on "being."

- Take care of their body (through healthy nutrition and exercise).

- Say, "I love you" often.

- Take risks.

- Say "NO" and get "feisty" (they say what they think and set boundaries).

- Prioritize freedom (they do what they want, not what they should).

- Live Mindfully – Be Here Now and Do it Now!

- Have an Attitude of Gratitude.

I do my best to live like this. You can live this way too; you don't have to wait for a cancer diagnosis!

Giving Thanks (on Thanksgiving)

Today is Thanksgiving Day, when the focus seems to be on food and all that we are going to eat.

Instead, today I find myself focusing on all that I am thankful for, mostly that I am still alive, happy, and (relatively) healthy, in my fourth year of living with Stage IV lung cancer. I seem to be beating the odds, and for that I am extremely grateful.

I am thankful for all my friends who continue to surround me with their love and support. I'm thankful for the presence of my younger son who is currently living with me, giving me all his love and support. I am thankful for my older son, my daughter-in-law, and my three amazing grandchildren who live so far away, yet always welcome me into their home; I'm so grateful that I can share in their lives whenever I can. I'm so thankful for my niece in Costa Rica and being able to share in her family when I visit. I'm grateful for my cousins who support me all along the way, and for my 92-year-old mother who continues to be a role model of living *her* life.

Of course I'm so grateful that I am getting the best possible medical care at Mass General Hospital; I'm sure my doctors are the best in the world.

I'm grateful that I have the energy and stamina to travel to exotic places (I just returned from Southeast Asia) and that I have the energy to go Zydeco dancing whenever I can.

While I didn't choose to get lung cancer, I am grateful that my diagnosis has helped me see what is most important to me: my family and friends and physicians. I start each day thinking about all that I am grateful for: it's *you readers*, in addition to all the others I have mentioned (see "Acknowledgments"). Thank you all for being in my life and for all that you do for me.

Happy Thanksgiving!

"Gratitude is not only the greatest of virtues, but the parent of all others." Cicero (106-43 B.C.)

The Best Present is Presence (at Christmas)

As I get caught up in all the stress of Christmas – what to buy for whom, how much to spend, letting people know what to buy me, I realize how unimportant all this stuff is, really. I have enough stuff; I don't need more. And I'm sure this is true for most of us. Years from now we won't remember the stuff we got, but we'll certainly remember the people we spent time with.

I get anxious about buying Christmas presents since I don't want to hurt anyone's feelings by giving the "wrong" present, or forgetting to give a present to someone, or not spending enough money on a present (unfortunately it sometimes seems that the value of the present represents the value of that person to you). It seems so silly to get anxious about all this.

What really matters during the holidays are the extra special connections to family and friends. Friends, especially old friends, make more of an effort to connect, as it's a great time to catch up on our lives. Families make more of an effort to get together, too. Christmas is often the only time I see both my sons and all my grandchildren at the same time. I love spending Christmas with my grandchildren, watching their excitement and enthusiasm. They love receiving their surprise presents, but I know they also love giving gifts that they have thoughtfully created. I get so much more out of *giving* than *receiving*. Most important for me, Christmas is about being with my grandchildren and my sons; it's more about **sharing my presence, not sharing my presents.**

I've recently been reading a lot about the concept of mindfulness, an important Buddhist principle that has us focus on the present moment in non-judging awareness and attention. Western psychologists have called it *present-centered awareness* or *unconditional positive regard.* Buddhism asserts that the very foundation of well-being is mindfulness. I really resonate with that and now, more than ever, I want to live my life as mindfully as possible.

Alan Watts says, *"The art of living consists in being sensitive to each moment, in regarding it as utterly new and unique, in having the mind open and wholly receptive."*

Another well-known quote says it well: *"Yesterday is history, tomorrow is a mystery, but today is a gift and that is why it's called the present."*

So for this Christmas holiday I am focusing on being mindful and being grateful for all the real gifts in my life, the *presence* of my loving family and friends. I will do my best to give them the most valuable gift I can: *my presence.*

My 50th High School Reunion

I recently attended my 50th high school reunion in La Jolla, CA. The 50th is *The Big One*. People seem to make more of an effort to attend, so I saw many people I haven't seen in over 50 years. It was really special to connect with those whom I shared so many experiences during my formative years. There's a certain comfort level that comes from these shared experiences and shared values. I felt home.

Actually, I think reunions are not so much about re-connecting with other people as they are about re-connecting with our self. It's the closest thing to time traveling; we turn back the clock and get in touch with whom we were *then*. People remember you the way you were then, too; they see the teenager in you under all the wrinkles and grey hair. That helps us see our teenage self also. People share memories of you (hopefully good ones) that were long forgotten. This is all part of our identity that stays with us as we age; my teenage self is still in me!

My reunion was bittersweet, actually, because I had left high school before we graduated. My mother took my sister and me with her to live in Spain when I was 14 (see "Gidget Goes to the Convent"). At the reunion of my high school class I could sadly see how much I missed by leaving. I think about all the "what ifs" had I stayed. Would I have been a cheerleader or a prom queen or a class leader? Would I have dated the popular boys? Would I have played a sport? Would I have been chosen as "best dancer" like I was later in the high school I finally graduated from? I'll never know. So, instead, I focus on all the positives of having attended, albeit so briefly, such a great high school in such a beautiful location. I'm grateful for the time I did have there (I'd been going to school with these same people since second grade). I'm grateful for the connections I made with some of those high school friends; many have been and will be lasting friendships.

I really did have fun at the reunion. At dinner we heard from each person in the class (over 75 of us) who did their best to sum up their life since high school. I was struck by how happy and successful most people seemed to be; there were many intact marriages. After dinner some of us danced to the "oldies but goodies," which also helped connect us to the feelings of the past. I was transported back in time while dancing with old boyfriends and old flames; I was a cute young teenager once again for that brief period of time. These are all happy memories to take with me to my deathbed; I will have a smile on my face every time I think of my 50th reunion.

Dancing in the New Year: 2013

Since being single I've always found New Year's Eve to be the most challenging night of the year. That's when being single is most poignantly felt; it's when I feel like a "missing half." I often feel lonely, but this year I didn't feel lonely at all. I danced (and danced and danced) into the New Year. Fabulous Fun!

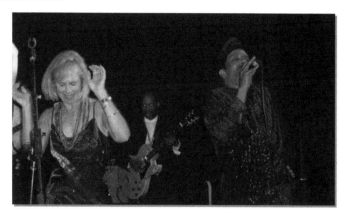

Dancing in the New Year

I was in Lafayette, Louisiana, with one of my best friends and dancing buddy, Francine, along with others who came from all over the U.S. and Canada. What a joyful way to greet the New Year: live music and Zydeco dancing. We actually spent five days (and nights) dancing; every day there were multiple venues, always with live Zydeco (and Cajun) bands. Each day brought unique and interesting and fun experiences (like celebrating New Year's Eve every day!). Some of the highlights include:

- Cafe des Amis: dancing during breakfast and out on the sidewalk (while standing in line).

- Whiskey River: a famous nightclub on the bayou, known for its live music and dancing (quite the scene, but really too crowded to dance).

- Club LA: an all African-American Zydeco club where we could experience the "real thing" (ending with a police raid).

- Dancing at the "World's Oldest Zydeco Club" with a mixed crowd of locals and out-of- towners.

- Club Vermillionville: dancing in the New Year with Francine and Mark (from Boston) to "When the Saints Go Marching In".

- Listening to a live Cajun music "jam" at a private home on New Year's Day with over a dozen world-class musicians playing guitars, violins, triangles, accordions… and singing.

Quite a few people from New England have moved to Louisiana permanently in order to dance all the time; I understand their passion. When I dance I feel totally in flow – totally in the moment. Everything else is forgotten as I connect with my partner; each connection creates a different energy and synergy (see "Why I Love Zydeco Dancing"). A dance can be an unforgettable peak experience; dancing fills me up and brings me joy. What better way to start the New Year!

What's my New Year's Resolution? You guessed it: keep on *Dancing Through Cancer*!

Living With Loss

Dealing With Loss

Living with cancer means living with loss.

When I recently wrote about dealing with the loss of my hair, I realized that the loss is much bigger than that. I've lost my body as I knew it; I've lost my identity (see "Loss of Identity: Who Am I Now?").

I've lost a part of my left breast; I've lost a lobe in my right lung (and a piece of the lower lobe); I've lost the normal functioning of my bowels; I've lost the normal texture of my skin and finger nails; I've lost a lot of weight; I've lost some clarity of vision and clarity of thought; I've lost my physical fitness; I've even lost my mind (see "Chemo Brain"). My body has become something different, but I am adjusting to the new *me*.

These losses have side effects: hiccups when I first eat; the more frequent need for reading glasses; constant yawning; occasional vomiting; frequent stomach cramps with unpredictable diarrhea; skin rashes, itchy dry skin, painful nail splitting and paronychias; dry mouth, dry eyes; extreme sun sensitivity resulting in raw lip burns; difficulty catching my breath when exerting myself aerobically, etc. (see "Managing Medication Side Effects").

The loss of my self-image – my identity – might be the most difficult to deal with: I am not the same person.

I've also lost my future as I knew it (see "Financial Planning").

But there is much about the new *me* that I like! In many ways my life has become richer and more meaningful. I have learned to appreciate what I have gained rather than what I have lost. I am more engaged and present and empathic; I live more in the moment; I appreciate the beauty of each day; I do my best to practice what the Buddhists call "mindfulness." Mindfulness is the ability to quiet the mind in order to sense the body and the world anew. It means listening to the crunch of snow on the winter path, hearing the wind in the trees, listening to the birds and bees, noticing the flowers, feeling the sun on my face. I try to **be here now**, and to be grateful each and every day for the richness of my life.

I am especially mindful of my relationships. I do my best to appreciate all the good things within people; I try to be less judgmental. I notice that my relationships have become much more intense and intimate. I appreciate having my friends and family in my life much more than I ever did; they are what matters most to me. I feel their love directed at and all around me. What a gift!

I have learned to put things in perspective; all my losses are minor in the grand scheme of things. I'm focusing on what is really important in life – I'm here and I'm loved! What can be better than that? I have certainly gained, not lost!

Loss of Identity: Who Am I Now?

Cancer has changed my identity; I'm a different person now. I think I'm a better person in many ways, but there are many things about myself that I do miss.

There have been many physical changes that I have had to adjust to and accept:

- I lost my long, straight, blonde hair, which I always thought was my best feature. Now my hair is short, dry and frizzy, and mostly grey. I don't think I look like the same person; I certainly don't feel as attractive (see photos).

- I used to be quite the athlete… in better shape than most of my friends. Now I can't exercise the way I used to; my physical ability is more limited. I huff and puff when I climb up a steep trail; I can't keep up while kayaking or biking or cross-country skiing with friends. I'm no longer an athlete. This is all very humbling.

- I have chronic eye problems due to dry eye. My eyes are always red and itchy and not very attractive.

- I have chronic stomach/bowel issues, which means making sure I am always near a bathroom. (For this reason alone I had to give up my work and identity as an Outward Bound Instructor.)

- I'm more dependent on others for help, and I need help more often. I've learned to ask for help and not feel needy.

- I'm much thinner; I'm a different body type. I've lost almost 30 pounds since my cancer diagnosis.

But I tell myself these are only physical changes, which are superficial. I think I've become a better person with all these changes because I've had to accept myself for who I am now. I look deeper within myself for my identity; I see myself from the inside, not the outside. I've learned to focus on what's important in life – relationships, leaving a legacy, and giving back. I've become more grateful and appreciative of the richness of my life.

How I look doesn't matter; what matters is how I feel and how I make others feel. I want people to feel touched by me and to remember me with love and respect. I make myself happy by doing my best to make others happy.

I like my new identity better. Who am I now? One identity I certainly don't want to have now is "cancer victim." My new identity is a more sensitive, caring person who focuses on enriching other people's lives, and as a result, enrich my own.

Losing Friends to Cancer

I just lost another good friend to cancer this month. It was unexpected and a total shock. I was traveling and heard about it through *her* email address, but the message was from her sister: "Sorry to inform you that my sister has died of cancer."

I couldn't believe it; I thought the email was a mistake. Not so. Apparently she had gone into the hospital because of some vague stomach pains; she thought she had an infection and just needed to cut back on her Advil® intake. Turned out she was full of cancer and died within four days.

I lost another good friend recently who died of complications with leukemia; this was also not expected (see "Facing Death").

I will miss them both immensely. They were special friends, Rheua Stakely and Vickie Ball, and I will always remember them. I like to think that a part of them will always stay alive within me.

It seems like cancer is an epidemic. Since my lung cancer diagnosis, there have been at least eight deaths from cancer among my friends; three or four more have been diagnosed with cancer. What is happening? Why can't we find better cures and treatment of cancer? It's scary and frustrating, puzzling, and maddening.

Of course, I was totally freaked out when I got my diagnosis, but I am doing okay for the moment. I seem to be one of the lucky ones who is managing to live with cancer. I am hoping I'm one of the 5% of advanced lung cancer patients who survive beyond the five-year mark. Those aren't great odds, but I seem to beating them so far.

When I was first diagnosed a friend said, "You'll probably outlive many people who are alive today." He was so right!

I'm reading the blog of another lung cancer survivor (Linnea: *"Life and Breath: Living with Lung Cancer"*) and I really resonated with her recent post:

"Cancer scared the shit out of me until I started living with it. Now it has become my new normal. Quite frankly, death is my familiar too. I've certainly thought a lot about my own mortality. And cancer has taken those I care about on a far too regular basis.

But, I now trudge willingly and without fear (a realistic dose of sadness is another story). It is my path and not without beauty. I've made the decision that I wish to be completely emotionally present; without any filters.

Having a terminal illness has given me access to an enhanced existence, as well as introduction to an amazing array of fellow travelers. We may have lost a bit of our innocence, but in turn we tend to travel light, be very clear-eyed and sure-footed, and share a tendency to seize every day. Our relationships quickly achieve an emotional intensity and intimacy that wastes little time, and in general we taste of life deeply. Truth, which does not avoid a very real connection to mortality, has set us free (I refer here not just to those with cancer, but to friends, family, and caregivers as well).

Death is an inevitable part of life and also a blessed release from suffering. If we can learn to embrace the journey, perhaps fear can be banished. And it is my goal to see it all with a clear head, to make the experience as full and rich as possible.

You don't have to have a cancer diagnosis to live a life as full and rich as possible. So I say: embrace the journey and seize the day!"

Thank you, Linnea, for articulating my similar thoughts and feelings so well!

The Environment

How Our Environment Affects Us

Our environment affects us immensely. What we look at, what we smell, what we hear, what we taste, what we touch, whom we are with; all this influences how we feel and what we think. People with SAD (Seasonal Affective Disorder) know quite well how the environment affects them; children living near noisy traffic areas are known to have poor concentration; suicide rates are higher for people in northern climates, and so on.

Feng Shui, the science of placement and proportion, is *the art of creating harmony and balance in your life by designing your environment*. Feng Shui experts say that if you move 27 things you will change your reality.

When I got my lung cancer diagnosis, I knew that I needed to change my reality (living in the city). I wanted to live in a natural environment, one filled with beauty and inspiration. I wanted a place that felt peaceful and relaxing; one that moved my spirit. I wanted a healing environment that reduced my stress while it stimulated me to live a fulfilling, meaningful life. I wanted to enjoy the outdoors each day. So I moved back to the ocean.

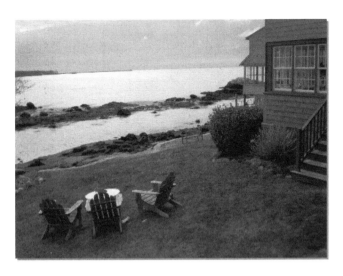

View From My Studio

I found the perfect little studio that overlooks the water in Gloucester, MA. Every morning in the summer I wake up to the sound of seagulls and ducks and robins and wrens. I sit outside, sip my coffee, feel the warm sun on my face, and smell the ocean. I watch sailboats and windjammers, even cruise ships, come into the harbor. I enjoy all the beautiful flowers and plants in my lovely yard. Later, I watch the magnificent sunset, and at night I relish the spectacular sky filled with so many bright stars (and sometimes a full moon). I go to sleep listening to the lapping of the waves as the tide goes in and out. Heaven on earth!

And the best thing about my environment is that my wonderful friends and community surround me! I am always with people who support, nourish, and inspire me.

Thomas Leonard, in his excellent book, <u>The Portable Coach</u>, states that there are two ways to perfect our environment: add to it or subtract from it. We can do things to enrich our life and we can do things to simplify our life. We need to live in places that we love, whether it's the ocean or the mountains or the farm or the city. Visually we need to create beauty inside, as well as outside our homes. Spiritually we need to create a space of peace and quiet in our life. We need to surround ourselves with sounds and smells that move us. We need to be with people who nurture and inspire us. We need to stimulate our minds with lifelong learning.

On the other hand, we need to reduce or eliminate stressors in our environment, like excess television and computer use, toxic people, clutter, unwanted noise, pollution, etc. This is easier said than done, but it's necessary if we want to be happy.

It is possible to choose and shape our environment to help us enjoy life to the fullest. We can be purposeful about it. I'm doing it the best I can, and I know my environment is helping me heal.

The Lazy Days of Summer

When summer comes to New England, I drop everything to enjoy it. I go outside every minute I can. (I feel conflicted now, as I write this blog while inside, since today is another beautiful, sunny day.) We in New England have had unusually warm and sunny days this year. California weather! I've been sailing in my sailboat in Ipswich Bay, kayaking off my back yard into Gloucester Harbor, swimming in a large private quarry, boogie boarding and stand up paddling in the waves at Good Harbor Beach, biking along the Back Shore, walking along the beach, hiking in the White Mountains, etc. – all with friends or family. What could be better? I am grateful that my health is so good that I can enjoy all this.

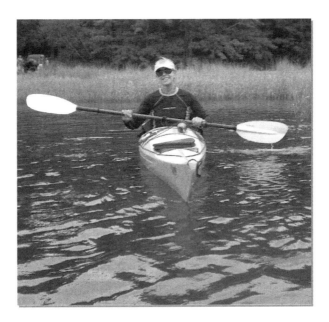

Kayaking

Exercising in the outdoors is such a treat. I purposefully live in an environment that is filled with beauty (see "How Our Environment Affects Us"). I de-stress the moment I go outside. I do my best to stay fit by balancing aerobic exercise with stretching and strengthening exercises. I do yoga; I also meditate; I get massages; I have done Reiki and Tong Ren Therapy (see "Tom Tam and Tong Ren Therapy"). I am doing all I can to heal my body (see "Healing Myself").

I don't have control over the cancer that has decided to take over my body, but I do have control over what I do to fight it. I take the recommended "miracle" chemo pill, Tarceva® daily; I eat a plant-based diet with minimal sugar and dairy; I surround myself with supportive friends and family; I try to live a stress-free lifestyle; I listen to music and I dance as often as I can; I exercise; and I try to have a positive attitude and to be grateful for what I have. I'm sure all this makes a big difference in my physical and mental fitness and healing. It's not just Tarceva® doing the work.

I know that one day I may not be so happy and healthy, but it feels like that day is a long way off. I plan to enjoy life now as much as I can by making the most of each day, being grateful for my current health and for the richness of my life.

Now I'm headed outdoors for some fun in the sun. I hope you're doing the same!

Not So Lazy Days!

Last post I celebrated the lazy days of summer and said that *not* being so happy and healthy was a long way off – *NOT!* I just spent five hours Saturday night in the Emergency Room of Martha's Vineyard Hospital dealing with a severe lip infection. I was given intravenous steroids and Benadryl® and Prednisone, and had to leave the island the next day in order to have an emergency consultation with a dermatologist at Mass General Hospital on Monday. It had to be determined if this new, more severe, lip problem was triggered by the Tarceva® (which causes extreme sun sensitivity). If so, I would have to go off the drug and, even more worrisome, I would then not be eligible for another clinical trial drug. This was a serious matter.

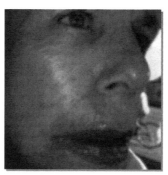

Infected Lips

After two days of doctor appointments and consultations, it was finally determined that what I have is a bacterial infection, not related to the Tarceva® (so now I go off the Prednisone and onto an antibiotic). This was really great news as I can continue with my Tarceva® treatment plan. Of course, I'm sure that the bacteria got into my lips because they were raw and swollen from the sun, so I must be even more careful when I'm outside (I always wear a wide-brimmed hat and even a face mask, but it wasn't enough this time).

This is one of the many challenges of taking drugs for cancer treatment: we never know what side effect is related to the drug. I have had a few other medical conditions (remember "costochondritis"?) since I've been on Tarceva® that have *not* been caused by it, but the Tarceva® effect always has to be ruled out. We never know. But the effects come and go, at least, and I learn to manage them.

It's hard not to get discouraged with all these medical interventions. I was in incredible pain and extremely worried and scared about what was happening in the hospital, but I got over it. I'll chock this up to another learning experience and keep my hopes up that Tarceva® will continue to keep the tumors at bay. In the end, that's what matters most.

The Joys of Travel

Creating Memories

I decided to move back to Gloucester, where I had lived for over 20 years and where most of my friends still live, so that I could be closer to them. I see friends every day now for walks and talks and more. I feel surrounded by love and support; this is priceless! And I fly out to California or Costa Rica or New York to see my family (mother, niece, grandchildren, sons, cousins) as often as possible.

Actually, what saddened me the most when I was first diagnosed was thinking that my grandchildren would not know me for very long. This is my greatest worry: that we will miss out on sharing life's events together. But I try not to think about that and, instead, focus on having good times with them whenever we're together, trying to make them as memorable as possible.

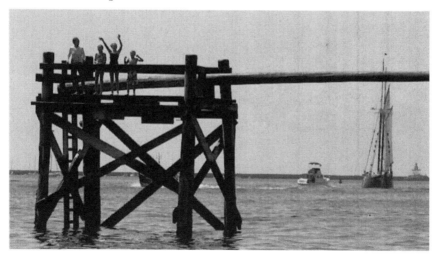

On the Greasy Pole with Grandchildren

One memory, during the summer when they were visiting me, stands out. They all (Madison, age 14; Taylor, age 12; Jack, age 9) wanted to swim out to the "greasy pole" in Gloucester Harbor (a greased up telephone pole placed horizontally on a platform that crazy, mostly inebriated men try to walk across in order to win the flag that is posted at the other end during St. Peter's famous fiesta in July). At first I didn't want to swim out there in the freezing cold water, but then I thought, "What a great memory this would be!" So my grandchildren and I all swam out, climbed to the top of the platform and then jumped off, shrieking and laughing. This experience is something we will never forget! And we have pictures!

I'm optimistic that we will make many more memories together.

Making More Memories

I just returned from California, visiting my mom (in Borrego Springs) and then my grandchildren (in Orinda). I just love seeing them. Spending time with them is my biggest priority and greatest joy right now, so I go out there as often as I can.

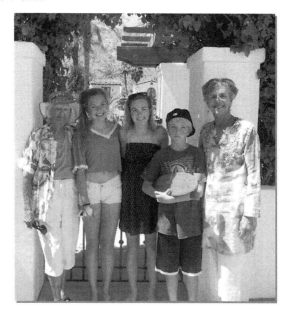

With My Mother and My Grandchildren

I'm so grateful that I get to share in their lives as often as I can; it's remarkable to see them grow and develop into interesting little people. Each one has her or his unique and special qualities, which I love to witness. I watch them in their various sporting events (softball, baseball, lacrosse, soccer, tennis, track, swimming, etc.), in other activities (school plays, music concerts, etc.), and interacting with their friends. On this visit I saw Taylor play softball, Jack play baseball, and Madison in her school play, "The Wiz." All of this was so wonderful to see! And I loved spending a fun family day with my son, Scott, and daughter-in-law, Lisa, and my grandchildren hiking in a beautiful park, and then eating out in a delicious restaurant.

I'm grateful to my son and daughter-in-law for inviting me to participate in their family vacations (Hawaii last spring; Bear Valley skiing after Christmas; Quechee, Vermont in the summer; and this Easter at their home). I always feel welcome with them. We're creating memories together, which is what is most important to me.

My legacy to my grandchildren is not leaving money or material things, but leaving them with fond memories (and this book) shared with someone who loved them dearly. I hope that they will feel I've made a positive difference in their lives and that perhaps I've given them different perspectives, viewpoints, and experiences that they might not have had. I'd like to think I've been a good role model or that I've enriched their lives in some ways. I don't remember much of my grandmother and for that I am sorry. I know Scott has fond, loving memories of his grandmother who died a few years ago. My hope is that his children, my grandchildren, will have the same fond memories of me.

I believe that our relationships shape us. In relationships, different aspects of ourselves are brought out that may have remained dormant, but that wake up in connection with someone else. Our relationships can open us up to new world views, different perspectives, and greater self-awareness. I hope that I can help bring out different aspects in my grandchildren through my relationship with them, which I hope will be for many more years. I also believe that my desire for being a part of their lives will keep me going for a long, long while!

California Dreamin'

I just returned from another visit to California where I go every three or four months to visit my mother, my son and his wife, and my grandchildren.

I grew up in La Jolla. I always love going there; it's part of my identity, my roots. I feel *home* when I'm there. La Jolla fills me up and connects me to myself. Even now, when people ask me where I'm from, I say, "I'm from California, but I live in New England" (where I've been for over 30 years). I hold on to my "California girl" image – my identity.

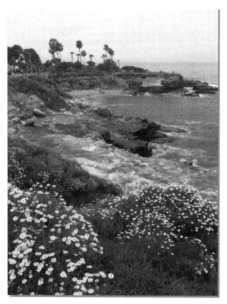

La Jolla Coast

Unfortunately, my mother left La Jolla and now lives in Borrego Springs (a beautiful desert community near Palm Springs, but far away from La Jolla). However, I always make time to visit La Jolla. My favorite cousin, Chrissy, still lives there, so I have a place to stay and a fun companion to do things with. Our favorite thing to do is walk the beaches from the famous Cove to the famous Windansea. The Cove is now an underwater park filled with colorful gold fish (garibaldis), lots of birds (pelicans, cormorants, sea gulls), seals, and now lots of sea lions. Once, we even saw a whale close to shore. There are also snorkelers, stand up paddlers, long distance swimmers, and many kayakers. Across the water there are hang gliders who soar off the cliffs of Del Mar. The spring flowers are amazing, all in yellows and blues and reds. I especially love the ice plant flowers and the delicious smell of the eucalyptus trees. We usually walk for about a mile along the coast, passing by the numerous seals that have taken over another beach, the Children's Pool. We walk on to Windansea Beach to watch all the surfers. Windansea is always mesmerizing with its frequent gigantic waves and spectacular sunsets.

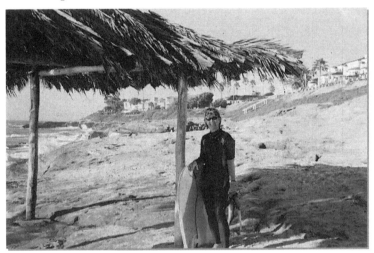

Boogie Boarding at Windansea

When I was a teenager I lived half a block from Windansea and played hooky many a day to go to the beach. Not to surf, however, because in those days the surfboards were way too large for a girl to manage. I guess I was a surfer groupie, like "Gidget." Sometimes I went out "tandem" with a surfer dude, so I learned how to swim in those big waves. Now I can ride those waves on a boogie board, but the young, male surfers don't really appreciate maneuvering around an old lady.

Perhaps I romanticize La Jolla a bit much. Maybe it's because my mother took me away from it when I was 14, an age when friends are the most important things in your life. She took my sister and me to Torremolinos in southern Spain and stuck us in a Spanish convent boarding school in Malaga. The culture shock was tremendous. I spoke no Spanish, I had barely ever been to church, and they separated me from my sister. I felt totally alone and bereft, and I cried every day (see "Gidget Goes to the Convent").

Sadly, I never went back to live in La Jolla, as I had hoped. My father, remarried and living in Virginia, wanted to pay in-state tuition for college, so I attended all-female Mary Washington College, and met my husband-to-be on a blind date. I transferred to the University of Virginia and married him. I followed him to New England, where he was from, and have lived here ever since.

However, I go to my LJHS reunions whenever possible; it's one way to reconnect to my roots (and old friends) and to get my La Jolla "fix." This year, in fact, was my 50th high school reunion (see "My 50th Class Reunion").

In a recent post I told about how I want to "make memories" with my grandchildren. I hope to share La Jolla with them some day soon, so that we can make that memory also.

I could return to live in La Jolla, of course, but I choose to live in New England (Gloucester) because I have so many wonderful friends here who nourish me and support me and care for me; I could never be without my friends. I think friends are the flowers and diamonds of life and are irreplaceable.

And I love my little studio overlooking the water, which nourishes me in a different way (see "How Our Environment Affects Us").

Also, my other son, Derek, now lives in Gloucester, so I get to spend time with him, which I cherish.

I feel like I have the best of both worlds. I'm so lucky!

Pura Vida (in Costa Rica)

My special niece, Liza, has made a wonderful life for herself in Costa Rica. Married to a "Tico", with an adorable toddler son, Felix (and now another son, Nico), she teaches/taught high school students at an international school. I visit her as often as I can manage – about once a year – and with each visit I discover more beauty in the country and I have more adventures. It's a country that has everything: beaches, lakes, rivers, jungles, hot springs, mountains, and beautiful flora and fauna. Costa Rica has recently been voted "the happiest place to live on earth."

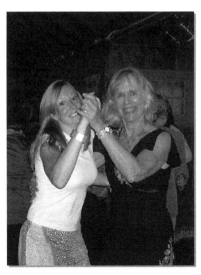

Dancing With My Niece, Liza

When I'm there I love feeling the warmth of the sun when I walk the beach and the warmth of the water when I swim in the Caribbean or the Pacific. I love seeing and hearing all the different birds (toucans, parrots, hummingbirds, and herons). I love the frequent sighting of monkeys (spider, whiteface, and howlers), sloths, turtles, snakes, and even crocodiles. I revel in the magnificence of the volcanic mountains, the banana and coffee plantations, and all the beautiful flowers. I enjoy eating the delicious fresh fruit and drinking fresh fruit juices every day. I always enjoy the sumptuous fresh vegetable dishes that my niece prepares.

I am even making connections with new friends and colleagues. When I visit, I always find time to volunteer at *Children's Well-Being Foundation*, a non-profit organization that provides life saving medical care and preventive health education to underserved families. I do what I can to contribute – translating, leading workshops, typing – whatever is needed. It feels good to give back a little and to try to make a difference in someone's life.

I also spend time with my new Tica friends whenever I visit, exploring San Jose and environs, finding new beaches, going out for lunch or dinner, and going salsa dancing. It's always an adventure!

And I have lots of opportunities to practice my Spanish. I like knowing that I'm keeping my brain active by speaking in another language.

The pace of life in Costa Rica is slower, so I always find time to read – to write – to knit – to meditate – to relax. And I love just hanging out with my grandnephew and seeing the world through his eyes. (see "Life Lessons From Babies").

There are always opportunities to be more active: to hike, to swim, to horseback ride, to go white water rafting or kayaking or surfing, or to explore the jungle.

I see my time in Costa Rica as healing and restorative and rejuvenating – bringing me peace and happiness while being with the people I love in such a beautiful natural environment. It certainly is *Pura Vida*!

Note: *"Pura Vida"* means literally "pure life" – and it is a common Costa Rican greeting to say hello or goodbye.

My Travel Bug

I think the love of traveling must be in my DNA. My mother always did a lot of traveling. Initially she planned to travel around the world in her 20's. She got as far as Hawaii (going west from California), married my dad, and two weeks later Pearl Harbor was bombed. That was the end of that journey! But she kept trying.

As children we traveled all over the place with our mother. We first lived in California, then Virginia, then back to California where we lived (in La Jolla, Del Mar, Alpine) until I was nine years old. Then my mother decided to move us all (my sister and brother and me) to Mexico City to live after she divorced my dad. However, we didn't stay long since we all got the measles and we needed to return to U.S. doctors.

When I was 11 she planned to move us all to live in Innsbruck, Austria, but she turned in the airplane tickets at the last minute because she had an opportunity to buy an affordable house near Windansea beach in La Jolla.

She tried again when I was 14. This time she took my sister and me to southern Spain. We stayed for two years in Spain (Torremolinos and Madrid) and one year in Germany (Munich). I returned for college in Virginia where my dad lived. By this time I had attended a different school almost every year.

When I was married we also moved around a lot: Rhode Island, New Hampshire, and finally settling in Massachusetts. We also lived in Puerto Rico for three years during my husband's Navy commitment. During our marriage, we took many trips to Europe, the Caribbean, and Asia.

The more I traveled, the more I wanted to travel. When I became single, I continued to do a lot of traveling with more trips to Europe, the Caribbean, Central and South America, and Southeast Asia. I'm also exploring new areas in the U.S.

All this moving around fostered my travel bug. I enjoy speaking other languages (I speak fluent Spanish, some French, and some German); I love getting to know other cultures; I love seeing and experiencing the beauty of other places; I delight in the food and drink of other countries.

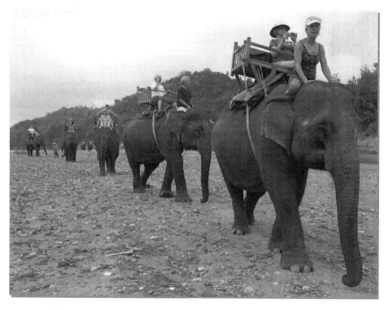

Riding an Elephant in Laos

I think traveling has made me a better person: I'm more sensitive to other cultures and people; I'm more appreciative of the beauty of my own country; I'm more aware of and value similarities and differences. I think I'm a more interesting person for having traveled so much. I'm more adaptable and flexible; I'm more accepting; I'm more cultured; I'm more knowledgeable.

Despite all the traveling I've done, I always seemed to have a big bucket list of places to go. However, my attitude changed dramatically when I got my cancer diagnosis. I realized, almost immediately, that traveling did not matter that much, really. All of a sudden, I didn't care about my bucket list. What mattered most to me is my relationship with my loved ones – my family and friends. If I have limited time on this earth, I don't want to spend it traveling to other countries *alone.* I want to spend my precious time with the special people in my life.

Now, if I travel, it is only when I am with family or friends. Ironically, I have been traveling more than ever. In the past couple of years I have gone on tours with friends to Australia and New Zealand, to Southeast Asia, to France, and Spain. My younger son and I spent a marvelous week together exploring Mexico City and environs. I just spent a fantastic week dancing in Louisiana with a friend (see "Dancing in the New Year: 2013"). Being able to combine my love of travel while sharing it with friends and family is an amazing gift; I am incredibly lucky and grateful. I'm also grateful that I feel well enough to travel.

My life will be shortened by cancer, so *each day matters.* My travel bug will just have to be dormant unless my friends or family come along – then I have the best of both worlds!

Gidget Goes to the Convent

(written in 1980)

One day I was your typical teenage California surfer girl living near Windansea Beach in La Jolla, and a month later I was stuck in a Catholic convent in Malaga, Spain, dragged there, along with my younger sister, by my divorcee mother looking for adventure. The culture shock was severe.

I was accustomed to the freedom of going out on dates, going to parties and after-football game dances, hanging out on the beach with my friends, and I had never even been to church! The convent allowed no such freedom – no dates, no dances or parties, no football games, no beach, and no friends. Instead we went to chapel three times a day (all day on Holy Days). We wore uncomfortable and unattractive uniforms with clunky shoes. We were allowed to take baths only once per week. No talking was permitted during meals, before breakfast, or on Holy Days. And, on top of all that, no one spoke a word of English, and I spoke no Spanish. I was miserable. I felt trapped and isolated, and homesickness engulfed me.

I experienced what it felt like to be a minority student. I was blonde and blue-eyed in a covey of girls with dark hair and dark eyes. They stared, pointed at me, whispered about me. I felt like a freak and cried every night in my little sleeping cubicle.

Eventually I adjusted. I learned to speak Spanish in a few weeks and could finally communicate as we sat over our embroidery in the garden (I had been placed in the "secretariada tract" since I couldn't speak Spanish well-enough for the "bachillerato" or "college" tract). Trini became my friend, a girl from a typical Spanish family, with twelve siblings. She opened my eyes to the beauty of Spain: Flamenco music and dancing, fiestas, Semana Santa (the

Easter week processions), paella, and bullfights. And, she introduced me to her brothers. When a young Spaniard serenaded me under my bedroom window while I was at home one weekend, I fell in love with the romance of Spain.

We stayed in the convent for six months, then traveled extensively through Europe, to eventually return to Spain – not to Malaga this time, but to Madrid, where I attended an American (Torrejon) Air Force Base school and graduated. Finally, after three years, I returned to the U.S. for college.

My experiences in Spain were very traumatic at times, but these experiences most definitely changed me in many positive ways. I know I am a different person from whom I might have been had I remained as "Gidget-on-the-beach" in California, which was made startlingly clear when I attended my 25th high school reunion years later.

What I Learned/Gained:

- Cultural Diversity: I developed a real understanding of a different culture, its language, religion, customs, and, especially, its people.

- Self-Confidence: I developed a greater understanding of myself through learning new skills and coping strategies. I like to think I turned adversity into opportunity and became a lifelong "climber" (from The Adversity Quotient by Paul Stolz).

- Awareness: I developed sensitivity to minorities that I think led in part to my social activism in the sixties' civil rights movement when I attended a Virginia college.

- Risk-taking: I learned new coping skills, developed new strengths, and found inner courage; all have served me well in other risking situations.

- <u>Spanish</u>: Speaking Spanish has brought me many new friends, exciting experiences, even professional work throughout my life.

- <u>A Role Model</u>: My mother followed her dream. She took her two daughters to Spain to reinvent her life and to have fabulous adventures. She showed me how to take risks that can lead to personal growth and to an exciting and fulfilling life. I have learned that it's possible to create the life you want. And I like to think that now I am a role model to my children, friends, and clients as I try to take responsible risks for personal growth and positive change.

Self-Healing – Alternative Medicine

Healing Myself

I am doing what I can to heal myself as I *dance through cancer.* While I have faith in western medicine and the treatment plan recommended by my oncologists at Mass General Hospital, I am also exploring and practicing alternative treatments. I think we all need to be our own health care advocates.

Here are some of the methods I am embracing:

- Diet – I've changed my diet drastically since my cancer diagnosis, now eating mostly a plant-based, organic diet, minimizing sugar and gluten. I also use a small amount of key supplements (Vitamins D, Omega 3, B12, along with a Pro-biotic). (I've written much about the rationale for this in many other posts on healthy eating.)

- Yoga – I practice yoga as often as I can. When I practice I feel stronger and more flexible, more balanced and centered, more relaxed and less distracted. I feel less stressed and I breathe better. Practicing the yoga postures are meant to awaken the body's chi – to get one's energy flowing by reducing blockages. Many studies point out the psychological, physiological, and spiritual benefits of yoga. Yoga is a great healing modality and I do my best to incorporate it into my life.

• Acupuncture – Many studies also point out the benefits of acupuncture, an ancient Chinese healing methodology. I found acupuncture to be very helpful in reducing my nausea when I was in the midst of chemotherapy infusion treatments. I also had monthly acupuncture treatments with Tom Tam (see "Tom Tam & Tong Ren Therapy") in order to remove blockages of energy – chi – to foster healing. I will use it again, as needed.

• Reiki – A coach colleague and friend, Grace Durfee (www.balancewithgrace.com), gifted me Reiki treatments during my chemotherapy regime. She used both "hands on" and "distance" Reiki. I definitely noticed benefits from her treatments, feeling less nauseous and more energetic. Like yoga and acupuncture, Reiki has been proven to remove blockages, increase energy and vitality, and boost the immune system, thus accelerating self-healing. Grace also trained me to use Reiki on myself. I have found it to be very helpful when I practice it.

• Massage – Massage has also been found to reduce blockages and promote energy flow for healing. I treat myself to a deep tissue massage as often as possible. Acupressure massages are also an essential part of Tom Tam's treatments, which I enjoyed.

• Meditation – After having gone to two meditation retreats, I am convinced of the value of meditation for self-healing. Meditation helps me feel less stressed and more relaxed, be more mindful and "in the present", and be less distracted. I'm sure that on my deathbed, meditation will help me feel more at peace (see "Committing to Meditation").

- Guided Imagery – Michael Samuels, in his book, Healing With the Mind's Eye, shares proven research and successful techniques for using guided imagery to heal the whole person – body, mind, and spirit. Guided imagery has been shown to reduce the side effects of chemotherapy and radiation in cancer patients. Patients who visualized healthy cells "eating" cancer cells often succeeded in reducing their tumors. When I meditate, I visualize the cancer cells being destroyed in my body. I'm optimistic that it's working!

- Exercise – Staying strong and vibrant is clearly important for health and healing. For that reason, I try to exercise as often as possible. I walk, bike, kayak, and ski with friends. I do a lot of dancing! I try to swim as often as possible, which, in addition to exercise, helps me breathe much better.

- Bibliotherapy – I've always been an avid reader: fiction, non-fiction, biography, and professional literature. Reading de-stresses me, educates me, distracts me. I enjoy discussing books with my monthly book group, "Inglenook." I know books help me heal.

- Stress – There is significant research that links stress to disease, especially cancer (see "Managing Stress"). I don't know if stress contributed to my cancer diagnosis, but I am doing my best to live stress-free now. I surround myself with loving and supportive friends. I spend as much quality time as I can with my sons and grandchildren and favorite niece. I minimize my contact with people who cause me stress. I only work when it's convenient, and I no longer do work that is stressful. I choose to live in a beautiful, peaceful environment on the water. I do everything I can for self-healing.

- Play – Play is an under-rated or un-appreciated activity; most adults stop playing when they "grow up." I think it is an essential activity to enhance one's quality of life; it is what gives life its passion and maybe even its purpose. I know how to play; I've always been good at it. I ski, sail, kayak, bike, hike, dance, travel, and much more. As an Outward Bound instructor, I helped people learn from play. Play fosters learning and healing so I plan to play as often as I can!

Many wise men have commented on the value of play:

- *"We learn more about a person through an hour of play or games than a year of conversation."* ~ Plato

- *"Everything we have learned in life we have learned by playing."* ~ Julio Olalla

- *"We do not quit playing because we grow old – we grow old because we quit playing."* ~ Oliver Wendall Holmes

- *"Play is one of the six most important skills/qualities for the 21st Century mind."* ~ Daniel Pink, author of A Whole New Mind

- Dancing – I've written much in many other posts about how dancing helps me heal. (See other posts on dancing).

- Nature – Being outside in nature has always felt healing to me; I try to get outside as often as I can. I moved back to Gloucester so that I can live on the water. I'm outside in the sun whenever possible. I sail and kayak and bike and walk and cross country ski outdoors whenever I can. Nature is definitely Nurture to me (see "How Our Environment Affects Us").

- Spirituality – Maybe what's most important for self-healing is to live a spiritual life. Lately I have been reading and studying Buddhism and its principles for leading a happy life. I am doing my best to live and practice these principles (see "My Spiritual Journey").

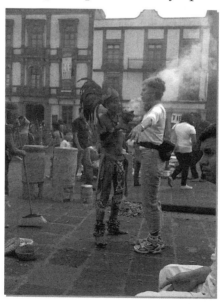

Getting Healed By a Curandero in Mexico

There are many other techniques to use for self-healing. A Chinese friend of mine (and lung cancer survivor) uses some unusual healing strategies learned from ancient China. All are designed to reduce or remove blockages in the body and to energize one's *chi*. Some examples are **slapping** your elbow, hand, knee, foot; **scraping** your arm with a smooth object; **"tiger point pressure"** (pressure point at base of thumb); **slamming** one's body against the wall; **sound healing** using **Tibetan Bowls**. I haven't tried any of these techniques, but his health has improved immensely since he started practicing them.

I think we all need to take responsibility for our own health and healing. I like to feel I have some control over my body, and that I may be able to foster greater healing than what is prescribed through my doctors. I then feel more empowered as I *Dance Through Cancer!* I also hope that the information in this book will help you learn how to become healthier and to feel more empowered.

Tom Tam & Tong Ren Therapy

Shortly after receiving my cancer diagnosis, a good friend suggested I see Tom Tam.

Tom Tam is a Chinese healer skilled at acupuncture and acupressure who is also a well-respected Qigong Master. However, he is most known for his Tong Ren energy healing, a therapy used for internally healing a patient's energy system, restoring health and vitality.

Tong Ren Therapy is based on the belief that disease is caused by blockages in the body's natural flow of *chi* (energy), thus it seeks to remove the blockages in a unique manner. A lightweight hammer is used to tap on the patient's targeted blockage points. However, the tapping is not done on the patient; it is done on a small human anatomical model (like a "voodoo" doll) as an energetic representation of the patient. The tapping is usually done in large groups with many dolls being tapped, capturing all the collective energy of the group to focus on one person at a time. Tapping can be done individually as well.

Tom Tam has had remarkable success curing people with terminal cancer, especially those for whom western medicine can no longer help. Many studies show that Tong Ren energy therapy can be an effective method for healing people with cancer and other serious illnesses. Once the blockages are removed, blood flow, neural transmission, and hormone reception are restored and the body is then able to heal. (For more, read Tom Tam's books: Walking Out of the Medical Jungle: Tong Ren Healing; or Tong Ren Therapy: What It Is, Why It Works, and How to Do It; or Tong Ren for Cancer.)

I saw Tom Tam in Chinatown many times for acupuncture and acupressure treatments, and I attended numerous Tong Ren groups led by him, as well as by others trained by him. However, I haven't seen him in over two years now as I have been doing so well. It's hard to determine what benefits I received from my treatments with Tom Tam since all along I have been following my western medicine protocol and eating a plant-based diet. So what is working? Of course Tom always thought my successful healing progress was due to Tong Ren Therapy. Who knows? The problem for many of us with cancer is determining what is working best to help us heal, since we often try multiple strategies at the same time.

I do know that if or when western medicine fails me, I will return to Tom Tam. It's nice to know he is there, continuing to produce miraculous healing. (For many of his success stories, read New Hope on the Horizon.)

Tom is becoming more and more respected and accepted in the western medical community, successfully leading his Tong Ren healing groups (called "guinea pig classes") at major Boston hospitals. Tom is also a prolific writer and poet so there is much to read about his unique approach to healing: <u>Tong Ren Healing: Guinea Pig Class</u>, also <u>Chi & Libido</u> or visit www.tomtam.com. He is also a frequent speaker, seen on television and *YouTube*.

It's important that those of us dealing with cancer become our own health advocate; we must take control, as best we can, of our own healing. We're lucky to live in a country where we have access to the best of western medicine, but it does not have all the answers. The more we can educate ourselves about alternative treatments, and actually practice them, the more options we have to help us live a longer life.

Nutrition

You Are What You Eat

I've become more and more convinced that we need to eliminate dairy and animal protein from our diets. Since my cancer diagnosis in 2008, I have been educating myself about healthy nutrition. The books I read, the documentaries I watch, and the workshops I attend consistently link dairy and animal protein with cancer. This information is based on solid research.

The good news is that we have control over what we put into our mouth; the bad news is that it's hard to control what we put into our mouth.

There is a lot of deliberate misinformation out there, so most people are confused about what makes up healthy nutrition. The dairy and meat industries work hard to foster this confusion, for obvious reasons. But the key information and true facts are out there.

If you watch "Food, Inc." you will see clearly the reasons not to eat meat and poultry: they are full of disease, steroids, and antibiotics (and corn!).

Watching "The Future of Food" or reading <u>The Silent Spring</u> will convince you to avoid eating any fruits and vegetables covered with pesticides, which means buy locally or buy organic.

The best new film out is "Forks over Knives." This is a must-see documentary revealing solid research linking animal protein to cancer, diabetes, heart disease, and more. (There are some amazing personal stories, too.) (For more film and book recommendations, see "Resources").

The choice to eat healthily is actually quite easy. It's just a little more expensive, sometimes hard to find organic food, and it takes more time to prepare. But what price health?

When I got my lung cancer diagnosis I immediately wanted to understand why I got it. I was not a smoker, nor had I lived in especially toxic environments, so what I had been ingesting into my body all my life seemed like a place to focus. At first I thought I needed to learn all about vitamin supplements (getting my nutrition in balance by understanding which vitamins to take daily). However, through my research, I became convinced that taking vitamins is not the answer; getting my nutrients through eating the right foods is the answer.

The best answer, actually, is eating a plant-based diet. Did you know that there is plenty of protein in green leafy vegetables? Also, that we really don't need as much protein as the FDA recommends. I make myself "green drinks" every morning (in my high speed blender, a Vitamix, I blend green leafy vegetables, like kale or spinach, with lots of fruit, fresh or frozen, along with coconut water or almond milk). I also make lots of fresh vegetable soups and veggie stir fries and super salads. I eat quinoa and tempeh and tofu, nuts and beans, hummus and carrots. There are so many choices!

My former dietary habits included eating meat every night with very little vegetables and almost no fruit. I ate lots of processed food; I loved cheese, milk shakes, sweets, and MacDonald's Big Macs! But I don't miss any of that now. And I don't feel deprived either, especially since I can feel the effect: I always have lots of energy all day long.

What about all those people, like my 92-year-old mother, who have lived a long life eating meat, dairy, processed foods, and sweets, and who are just fine? They seem to prove the point that what we eat doesn't matter. All I can say is, they're lucky. We know that 30% of smokers will get lung cancer, which means 70% won't, but why take the chance that you will be in the 30% (remember, 15% of non-smokers will get lung cancer)? As time goes on I'm certain more and more studies will show the link between cancer and animal protein / dairy / processed foods.

Study after study shows a higher rate of disease caused by eating "poorly." Why take that chance? It's within your control; it's your choice.

Do yourself a favor and educate yourself about healthy eating, then decide. I feel certain you will choose health.

See "Resources" for more films, books, and websites.

What I've Learned About Healthy Nutrition

Our bodies are still made to eat and move the way our Paleolithic ancestors did more than 10,000 years ago, yet we eat and move very differently now. We are paying a very high health price. Chronic diseases (cancer, diabetes, heart disease) are increasing; obesity is rampant. Paleolithic wo/man ate no dairy, no sugar, no gluten, and no oil; there were no processed foods. They ate mostly fruits and vegetables, nuts and seeds, fish and shellfish, and, surprisingly, very little meat.

Our diet today is 75% non-paleo and it is killing us. The average American diet includes only about 5% fruits and vegetables (which should be at least 50% of our daily intake). 60% of our food is processed; we ingest about one-third of a pound of sugar per day and about 8,000 mg of salt (our bodies only need 300 mg per day). We only eat 8-11 grams of fiber per day (paleo wo/man ate 110 grams per day). And, of course, we get a lot less exercise than our ancestors.

Seventy percent of our diseases are caused by our poor life choices (diet and exercise and stress), yet most of us are confused about how to eat healthily.

I hope the following information helps clear up some of the confusion. Here are some common questions (and answers)...

What's wrong with animal protein?

- Neu5gc is a unique sugar, found in meat, which causes rapid cell turnover. We are the only mammal that doesn't have this nutrient, having lost it about 20,000 years ago. Other mammals need this nutrient for accelerated physical development so that young livestock can walk or run a few hours after birth. However, they have a much shorter life span. Like humans, birds and reptiles, and most fish (except for salmon) don't have this nutrient. When we eat meat and dairy we are ingesting neu5gc, thus increasing cell turnover, which also leads to inflammation, autoimmune conditions, tumors, and cancer.

- IGF-1 (Insulin-like Growth Factor), found in animal protein, also accelerates the growth of normal tissue, as well as diseased tissues like cancer. Therefore IGF-1 accelerates aging. Calves need this to grow to 600 lbs. in six months; humans don't need to grow like that!

- Acidic vs. Alkaline diet. Animal protein increases the acid load in our body; an acidic environment fosters cancer growth. A high alkaline diet is much healthier.

- Cholesterol is found nearly exclusively in animal products. Cholesterol contributes to heart disease; it also facilitates cancer development.

- Methionine, a sulfur-containing amino acid found mostly in animal protein, metabolizes into homocysteine, which is a known risk factor for heart attack, stroke, dementia, depression, and more.

- Non-organic meat and poultry are full of antibiotics, disease, steroids, and corn (watch "Food, Inc." for more detailed information).

What's wrong with dairy?

- Casein: T. Colin Campbell, in his famous research, The China Study, found that casein, a protein found in 87% of dairy, caused tumors in mice 100% of the time! The mice that had tumors lost them when casein was removed from their diet. Also, cancer cases in China were found only in the affluent areas (where people could afford to eat or drink dairy). Some studies also show a positive correlation of casein with heart disease, Type II diabetes, and increased LDL.

- Cancer is caused, at least in part, by both high-and low-fat dairy products, according to Dr. John McDougall in The Starch Solution.

- Neu5gc and ICF-1 are also found in dairy.

- Non-organic dairy is also full of steroids, antibiotics, arsenic, disease, etc. Dairy products have been the foods most often recalled by the FDA because of contamination with infectious agents such as salmonella, E.coli, bovine leukemia virus, etc.

What about getting enough calcium?

We can get our calcium from sources other than milk, for example, green leafy vegetables, tofu, fish, green tea, and fruit. Silica (cabbage, kale, bok choy) is the best source for improving bone strength, as is Vitamin D. Bone strength and retention is more related to mineral retention than to calcium intake. We actually don't need as much calcium as we think.

Interesting fact: populations that consume the most cow's milk and other dairy products have among the highest rates of osteoporosis and hip fractures in later life (from the *British Journal of Medicine*, 2006). There are countries that have no osteoporosis and they drink NO milk (read The Starch Solution or The Blue Zone).

And don't forget that physical activity – especially weight bearing and strengthening exercises – is also critical in maintaining bone mass.

What about getting enough protein?

We can get protein from sources other than meat, for example, soy, tofu, tempeh, quinoa, green leafy vegetables, fish and shell fish, beans and legumes. We actually don't need as much protein as the Recommended Daily Allowance (RDA). (To determine your daily protein needs, multiply your weight in kilograms times .8 = grams). Vegan proteins may reduce the risk of cancer, obesity, and cardiovascular disease by promoting increased glycogen activity. Since plants contain sufficient protein and calcium for large animals (elephants, horses, cows, even dinosaurs), humans can certainly get all the protein they need through plants!

What's wrong with gluten?

A high gluten diet (breads and grains and cereals) can lead to arthritic-like symptoms, allergies, digestive ailments, and bone loss, even dementia. When presented with gluten, the cells that line our intestines have an immune reaction that produces inflammation and leads to a heightened autoimmune response.

What about supplements?

The problem with supplements is knowing how to balance them – knowing what supplement works well with what other supplements, as well as what supplements *your* body needs and in what dose. It all seems very complicated. It's easier to just eat your nutrients. The only supplements we really need are Vitamin D (those of us who don't get enough sun exposure) and Vitamin B12 (which is only found in meat).

How can I have a healthy diet?

- Eat large amounts of fresh green leafy vegetables and fruits (should be half of your plate) daily.

- Restrict or eliminate animal protein and dairy. Instead, drink soy, almond, hemp, or rice milk; eat soy or goat or sheep yogurt and cheese, instead of cow milk, yogurt, and cheese.

- Eat organic and local whenever possible.

- Restrict sugar and salt consumption (watch: "Sugar: The Bitter Truth" on YouTube)

- Restrict gluten-based flours; instead eat quinoa, buckwheat, millet, or amaranth.

- Eat brown or wild rice rather than white rice; eat sweet potato rather than white potato.

- Eat more nuts and seeds, beans and legumes.

- Get outside into the sunlight more often (at least 15 minutes per day without sun screen).

- Exercise a lot more! Get up and move around after every hour of sitting. Paleo wo/man spent about 12 hours each day exercising; the average person now spends about ½ hour each day exercising.

- Watch any of the movies and read any of the books I've listed in "Resources" for more information.

- See other posts on nutrition.

- Check out John Bagnulo's website: Terra Madre Farms, filled with articles and information. I learned all this information from his lectures and consultations.

Food as Medicine

Yesterday I attended a conference, "Cancer in the Family: Living with Uncertainty," at Massachusetts General Hospital. This is the third annual conference, all of which I have attended (see "Living With Cancer - Navigating the Cancer Journey"). I always learn a lot about recent research and more (see "Facts and Information (What I've Learned So

Far"), but mostly I felt inspired and supported and hopeful being with other brave souls who are managing to live with cancer.

However, I am always appalled at the food that is served! I complained about it last year, and this year it was no better. For breakfast we were served all sugary foods: sweet rolls, Danishes, bagels with jams and cream cheese. No fruit. Lunch had few vegetarian options and, by the time I got there, the vegetables were all gone. I ate a salad of iceberg lettuce and little else.

It seems so contradictory for a hospital to present a conference that's meant to help cancer survivors, yet serve food that may actually foster cancer. Much research shows that cancer loves sugar. For instance, a recent "60 Minutes" episode (April 2, 2012) graphically demonstrated this: P.E.T. scans are used to find cancer in the body by injecting a sugar-like substance because cancer cells light up when they come in contact with the sugar. Dr. Lustig gives a very thorough explanation about the toxicity of sugar in our diets on *YouTube*: "Sugar: The Bitter Truth." Dr. Mark Hyman, in his new book, The Blood Sugar Solution, gives a complete analysis of the dangers of sugar in our diet.

People go to hospitals to heal; yet the food most hospitals serve their patients does not promote healing – in fact much of the food practically promotes disease. This must change!

I don't understand why the medical community never addresses nutrition as part of the equation when it comes to health and healing. In one of the presentations yesterday about "sporadic cancers" (those that are not genetic), the speaker listed the contributors to lung cancer as environmental, smoking, and "other." Why was nutrition not on that list? Nutrition is a big contributor to our health. People need to be educated about healthy nutrition: what to eat and what to not eat. It's clear that our diets are killing us;

just look around. Obesity, heart disease, Type II diabetes, and cancer are rampant, and it's getting worse.

There has been a lot of research over the years about the role food plays in health and disease, and there are many integrative doctors successfully treating cancer patients with healthy nutrition. Thousands of patients have been helped and healed by following a healthy nutrition program. Yet the majority of physicians and hospitals don't recognize this factor; nutrition is rarely part of the equation for treating cancer or other diseases. Steve Jobs noted that "nutrition is not addressed in relation to oncology and pain care."

Why is nutrition never part of a health care regime? It's because doctors really don't know much about nutrition; medical school training includes very little nutritional education. A bigger reason, sad to say, is probably money. There is no motivation to incorporate "food as medicine" when drugs feed the pharmaceutical and medical industries. This needs to change! But I think change will have to come from grass roots efforts; each of us needs to demand that food as medicine be part of our treatment plans. We also need to educate ourselves about healthy eating (see "What I've Learned About Healthy Nutrition"), which mainly means eating a whole food, plant-based diet including fruits and vegetables, nuts, seeds, and beans; avoiding dairy; minimizing gluten; and eliminating sugar and all processed foods. There *are* delicious alternatives to our current poor diets (see "Suggestions for Healthy Eating").

Of course not all the blame goes to hospitals and the medical community. Our food is becoming less and less nutritious as agriculture objectives in the past 60 years have been for greater yields, faster maturation, greater resistance to bruising and damage, and longer shelf life. The dairy and meat industries have powerful lobbies and advertising; processed food is big business. (If you want to read more about the control big business and pharmaceuticals have over food production and sales, watch "Food Matters" or read The China Study.)

I hear people say there isn't enough research or proof that food may contribute to disease. I never understand that viewpoint, as there are many articles, books, films, and websites that document the results of successful alternative treatments and current research about healthy eating.

John McDougall, in his new book, The Starch Solution, makes it crystal clear, with vast supportive research, that a plant-based diet is the only healthy way to eat.

T. Colin Campbell, author of The China Study, showed the link between dairy and cancer and other diseases through his groundbreaking research.

Kris Carr, in her book, Crazy, Sexy Cancer, tells her personal story of surviving an extremely rare sarcoma called epithelioid hemangioendothelioma (EHE) by eating only a plant-based diet. She was only given a few months to live; yet nine years later she is alive and well.

Dr. Servan-Schreiber, M.D., diagnosed with brain cancer, extended his life by years by mostly following a plant-based diet. He wrote about his experience in Anti-Cancer: A New Way of Life.

Rip Esselstyn wrote The Engine 2 Diet because of the success he and his fire-fighting buddies had in drastically reducing their cholesterol levels by incorporating a plant-based diet.

And let's not forget the one who started it all, Frances Moore Lappe, with her groundbreaking book, Diet for a Small Planet.

The book list goes on and on… (see "Resources").

There are many physicians who are having great success curing cancer by mostly prescribing a plant-based diet to their patients. Here are a few of them:

Dr. Gerson claimed he cured cancer back in the 1940's. The Gerson Clinic continues to cure cancer patients today by using a severe nutritional therapy regime. Who has heard of him? For some reason their clinic has to be in Mexico since the U.S. does not allow nutritional therapy treatment in our country! For more information about the Gerson clinic, watch "The Gerson Miracle" or "The Beautiful Truth."

Dr. Nicholas Gonzales, of New York, has also had a lot of success with his treatment protocol, which is mostly based on a healthy diet of fruits, vegetables, and plant foods. What's wrong with our health? According to Gonzales, *"wrong diet, not enough nutrients in the food we eat, coupled with a lot of environmental exposures, and you get the present cancer epidemic."* You can read more about him in Suzanne Somers' book, Knockout: Interviews With Doctors Who are Curing Cancer and How to Prevent It In the First Place.

Dr. Caldwell Esselstyn, a former cardiac surgeon at the world-renowned Cleveland Clinic, reversed heart disease by having his patients adopt a whole-foods, plant-based diet. He describes his research in The China Study.

There are many more doctors and researchers with similar success stories, for example, Dr. Dean Ornish, Dr. Neal Barnard, David Wolfe, Andrew Weil, and many more.

Some films well worth watching include:

"Fat, Sick, and Nearly Dead" – two very over-weight men (350 and 430 lbs.) lose their weight (both drop to 200+ lbs.) and become very healthy by juicing with green plants and fruits.

"Food Matters" – This ground-breaking documentary sets about uncovering the trillion dollar worldwide "sickness industry" and exposes a growing body of scientific evidence proving that nutritional therapy can be more effective, more economical, less harmful, and less invasive than most conventional medical treatments.

"Hungry for Change" - This documentary empowers and provides practical and realistic solutions to healthy nutrition.

"Forks over Knives" – This documentary examines the profound claim that most, if not all, of the degenerative diseases that afflict us can be controlled, or even reversed, by rejecting animal-based and processed foods.

"Food, Inc." – This documentary shows how our cattle and chickens are raised, squished in a feedlot or a window-less building, fed only corn, ingested with antibiotics and steroids.

"Fast Food Nation" – This documentary shows how we all are affected by the fast food industry and the real and disturbing flaws that exist in meatpacking plants.

"The Future of Food"; "How to Cook Your Life"; "Supersize Me"; "Vegucated" are more movies I recommend about nutrition and food.

More doctors need to heed these wise words from Thomas Edison: *"The doctor of the future will no longer treat the human frame with drugs, but rather will cure and prevent disease with nutrition."*

Until then, we must be our own doctor!

Suggestions for Healthy Eating

Eating healthily is really not all that difficult. You just plan ahead a little, making healthy substitutions and good choices. And it can be really fun to find new recipes and new ways to cook. The following suggestions are ideas on how to eat the "Paleolithic way" – a plant-based diet excluding meat, dairy, sugar, and gluten.

When Traveling:

- Buy a salad in the airport; add an envelope of tuna or a can of sardines on to it. If you order a Caesar salad, ask for anchovies on it, and don't eat the croutons.

- Take along an apple, pear, orange, avocado, nuts.

- Bring a small bag of hemp protein to add to a fruit smoothie. When at home, make your own smoothies or juices (mix greens with fruit) to take with you in the car (for lots of recipes, read <u>Crazy, Sexy Juices & Succulent Smoothies</u>, by Kris Carr).

- Eat sushi made with brown rice.

- Make a gluten-free sandwich (almond butter, tuna, or egg salad) to go.

- Mexican food can be healthy: bean burritos, fish tacos, huevos rancheros, refried beans, guacamole, and veggie fajitas.

Substitutions:

- Avoid bread – instead, eat gluten-free bread, rice crackers, corn or rice tortillas.

- Avoid sugar – eat fruit instead.

- Avoid dairy – that includes cheese (if you must, eat dairy, choose goat or sheep products). Instead, drink soy, almond, or rice milk.

- Eat brown or wild rice instead of white rice – better yet, eat quinoa.

- Eat sweet potato instead of white potato.

- Instead of oatmeal in the morning, eat hot quinoa with fruit and nuts.

- Have buckwheat pancakes or waffles (with blueberries) instead of white flour pancakes or waffles.

- For sweetener, use local honey – minimize maple or agave syrup.

- Use veganaise instead of mayonnaise; Earth Balance® instead of butter.

- Use only extra virgin olive oil or coconut oil for cooking; avoid safflower, canola, etc.

- Drink your coffee black or, better yet, drink green tea.

- Eat whole oranges and grapefruit instead of drinking the juice.

- Eat only organic peanut butter or almond butter or cashew butter.

- Instead of white or wheat flour, use whole grain buckwheat flour – garbanzo bean flour – fava bean flour – almond flour – rice flour – amaranth.

- Healthy snacks include nuts like almonds, Brazil nuts, mixed nuts; hummus with carrots, celery, or cucumber; organic peanut butter or almond butter on celery or on an apple or pear; fresh fruit, avocado.

- Instead of meat, eat shellfish (especially oysters), fish (avoiding swordfish and raw tuna), and be sure to eat only wild fish, never farm-raised.

- Eat tofu and tempeh.

- Eggs – best to eat soft-boiled or poached or "over easy" (eat the eggs on top of cooked spinach or mushrooms); when baking, use only egg whites.

- If you must eat meat or chicken, make sure it's pasture-fed, preferably local.

- Eat organic and local as often as you can.

If interested, go to www.Kripalu.org for some great healthy recipes, or see a list of recipe books in "Resources".

Spring Deep Clean

Since my cancer diagnosis four years ago, I have been educating myself about food and what really is healthy nutrition. I may have no control over the cancer cells, but I do have control over what I eat or don't eat. I have learned a lot (which I share in different posts: "You Are What You Eat" or "What I've Learned About Healthy Nutrition").

Last week I went on a five day retreat at Kripalu, a yoga center in western Massachusetts, to learn even more about nutrition and to "de-tox" my body. There were 40 of us from all over the U.S. John Bagnulo, Ph.D., MPH, was our extremely knowledgeable, charismatic leader/teacher. We ate only fruits and vegetables – no sugar, no grains, no gluten, no dairy, no nuts & seeds, no coffee, and no alcohol. We hiked and practiced yoga each day following a two-hour lecture on nutrition. The purpose of this regime was to clear toxins out of our liver and kidneys, re-set our taste buds, and reduce our addictions.

The results for many people were quite remarkable. I, for one, cleared up my chronic sinus problem; no more post-nasal drip! My friend eliminated severe arthritic-like symptoms in her elbows (we believe that eliminating gluten is what cured us both!). Another woman got rid of a chronic coated tongue and bad breath (from eliminating dairy). A man struggling with high blood pressure now finds it to be in a consistently normal range. Everyone lost weight. I've also noticed that I feel much clearer in the head in the morning, not being in my usual "fog."

Once we finished the program we were encouraged to go on a "Paleolithic" diet: continuing to eat lots of fruits and vegetables, adding nuts and seeds, beans and legumes, brown or wild rice, quinoa, buckwheat, or millet; also fish and shellfish. Minimal meat and no dairy or sugar.

Many research studies link animal protein, dairy, and sugar to chronic diseases like Type II diabetes, high blood pressure/hypertension, and cancer. I've read that 70% of our diseases are caused by our life choices. I don't choose to eat anything that will feed the cancer cells in my body, so I plan to avoid sugar, meat, and dairy as much as possible. I will also stay off gluten longer since I feel so much better.

Acceptance and Attitude

It's All About Attitude

People are always telling me I have such a positive attitude (considering that I am living with Stage IV lung cancer and am dealing with all the difficult side effects of chemotherapy). I always say, "Why would I choose to have a negative attitude and feel miserable? I'd rather choose to be happy." We all have a choice on how we look at the world; we create our perceptions of reality. So, why not create perceptions that foster a positive attitude?

In another post, I wrote about stress and its impact on health. I believe that our attitude is the key component to effective stress management (see "Managing Stress").

Recently I had a great lesson in attitude adjustment. While in California I had made a plan to visit a former dance instructor who is living with late-stage lung cancer. The day of our date something came up and I had to cancel at the last minute. I felt terribly guilty; I expected him to be annoyed, frustrated, and even angry. His reaction was remarkable. He said, *"I am definitely calm and relaxed about missing your visit, because it is part of life and you have given me another lesson on missing opportunities. It does not mean that I am missing life. Just not all the parts are going with my plan, but some other higher power's plan! So you have already helped me without knowing it."*

What a lesson I learned from him! I let go of my negative judgment of myself: I forgave myself and learned, once again, how we create our reactions. We can choose to be stressed and anxious and annoyed and angry and guilty, or we can choose to be understanding, compassionate, forgiving, and grateful. It's not easy; it takes practice. My friend helped me learn a lot this time; he gave me a huge gift, for which I will always be grateful. And next time you encounter a stressful situation, I hope you will think of my friend and be reminded that *you* choose *your* reaction to stress. Choose positively!

Many famous people have remarked upon the power of our thoughts with the following quotes:

"There's nothing so upsetting in life, but thinking makes it so." ~ Shakespeare

"I am the story I tell myself I am." ~ Victor Frankl

"No one can make you feel inferior without your consent." ~ Eleanor Roosevelt

"People are about as happy as they make up their minds to be." ~ Abraham Lincoln

"What disturbs people's minds is not events, but their judgments on events." ~ Epictetus

"Psychological stress resides neither in the situation nor the person; it arises from how the person appraises an event and adapts to it." ~ Lazarus

"Stress is neutral - it is our reaction to it that determines whether it will be beneficial or harmful." ~ Hans Selye

Quotes worth remembering!

The Blame Game

The first question people ask when I tell them I have lung cancer is – you guessed it – "Were you a smoker?" I guess if I were to answer "yes" to this question then maybe it would somehow justify my diagnosis, like I was to blame or somehow I deserved this. There is a real stigma around the one cancer that causes more deaths than any other cancer: lung cancer. Why is that? I think people are trying to find reasons why *they* will never get lung cancer: if they never smoked, they're safe. But, sorry to scare you, about 40% of lung cancers occur in people who have already quit smoking, and 15% of lung cancer victims were non-smokers.

We do know that smokers are 30% more likely to get lung cancer, but the question that is missed by all of the statistics is: *Do smokers really deserve their cancer?* Most smokers of my generation didn't know the dangers of smoking and became addicted before it was too late to stop. It took a lot of strength and courage to quit, but most of my friends finally did. (None of them have developed lung cancer, by the way.) And what about all the smokers who never get lung cancer? Why not? All the causes of lung cancer are still unclear and, unfortunately, not enough research is being done to clarify the confusion. The statistics for lung cancer deaths have not changed over the years, whereas those for breast cancer have changed significantly. We do know that research can make a big difference in extending the lives of cancer patients.

Why is it that lung cancer patients are the only cancer victims who are blamed? Women diagnosed with breast cancer are never blamed, nor are people diagnosed with leukemia or pancreatic or prostate or colon cancer, etc. Obese people who get heart attacks or strokes are not blamed. Why is it that society blames only those diagnosed with lung cancer? Like somehow they brought it on themselves. Sadly many former smokers who get lung cancer blame themselves also; so they must live with guilt along with the stigma and pain of lung cancer. It reminds me of when I was working on a rape hotline and how rape victims were so often blamed ("Why were you out so late at night?"). I think when people *blame the victim*, they are really seeking a rationale that will leave them safe ("I would never go out so late alone at night." "I never smoked. Therefore I will never get lung cancer.") Think again! Statistics disprove these rationales. And, besides, if you have lungs you can get lung cancer!

So how do they (we) get lung cancer? I don't think anyone knows for sure, but here comes the self - blame part: **What did I do to foster lung cancer?** Did I consume too much sugar (I *love* desserts) over the years? Did I eat too much dairy - cheese - meat - processed food - fried food - Big Macs? Did I not eat enough vegetables and fruit? Did I allow too much stress in my life (see "Managing Stress")? Did the few cigarettes (and pot) I smoked cause it? Am I like the virgin who gets pregnant on her first sexual experience? I do blame myself for all this, but I also do my best to forgive myself.

The reality is that somehow I got lung cancer, so now I have to deal with it. Now I know what a healthy diet is, so I do my best to follow it; I live as stress-free as possible; I follow doctors' orders. I surround myself with supportive friends and family and I live in a beautiful environment that nourishes me each day.

This blame-game is really not helpful nor productive. It does nothing to foster positive healing or sensitive support. Smokers don't deserve to be blamed any more than non-smokers do. Better to focus on healthy, stress-free living as best we can. We're all in this together. We're all going to die of something sometime, so let's make this journey as healthy and happy as we can while we're on it.

The Black Box

I look healthy. I have loads of energy. I feel well. So it's easy to forget that I have metastatic lung cancer. I forget and my friends and family forget; people who first meet me are shocked when they find out about my illness.

I guess it's mostly a good thing to forget. I can focus instead on all the positives in my life and enjoy each day. Then I feel good. Why focus on cancer? Then I feel bad.

But the reality (cancer) is always there, like a dark cloud hanging over my head or an ax waiting to fall. Recently I met with a new oncologist who said we need to acknowledge the unique stress of living this strange dichotomy: looking and feeling good while living with a progressive terminal illness. She said it's like having a black box that one keeps on a shelf, filled with fears and anxieties, sadness and anger, guilt and regrets. It's always there and best to keep it closed, but it must come down and be opened once in awhile for a reality check. Maybe it's like not ignoring "the elephant in the room." Maybe more stress is created if it is ignored. Maybe if I open the box once in awhile and face the reality of my situation, then I will live my life more purposely and mindfully. I will appreciate the preciousness of life.

The reality of cancer puts one face-to-face with death (see "On Facing Death"). But knowing that death may come sooner than expected helps one (me) realize what's most important in life and to prioritize my actions. So I do my best to live each day focusing on my priorities: my family and my friends.

So I'll keep the black box on the shelf for as long as I can, knowing that taking it down once in awhile is okay and a helpful reminder to always live fully and lovingly.

You Look Great

People tell me this all the time, but I have mixed feelings about it. I know I don't look like I have cancer, and people are surprised that I don't look the way they think a cancer victim should look, but I have Stage IV metastatic lung cancer! Cancer is often an invisible disease; illnesses that are invisible can be harder to live with in many ways.

Why does it bother me that I'm told I look great? In some ways it feels dismissive, as if people don't want to talk about cancer. It doesn't give me a chance to talk about what's concerning me about how I'm feeling *today*. It closes the conversation.

It's disconcerting when someone who "looks healthy" is diagnosed with a serious illness. This situation strikes fear in all of us because being healthy is supposed to protect us from disease. When someone who looks healthy is really very sick, it can make us feel vulnerable, so we don't want to talk about or acknowledge it. We look for reasons why it would never happen to us (which I think is why so many people ask me if I ever smoked). I call this "blame the victim" syndrome. The belief is: *"If I didn't or wouldn't ever do that, then maybe I'll be safe."* When someone is stricken down for no explainable reason, it's frightening; we think, "Oh my god, it could happen to me!" So people look for a reason to blame the victim.

What do I want people to say to me? Just ask me how I'm feeling or how I'm doing today; let me talk about what's on my mind. Or tell me what you appreciate about me, specifically. Or just listen. Just *be* there; your *presence* is really all I need. Show me that you love me. They say that non-verbal communication is two-thirds of the conversation, so you don't need to *say* encouraging words in order to communicate support and caring and unconditional love.

These would also be some of the same things to say to someone who is close to death. Yalom, in his book, <u>Staring at the Sun: Overcoming the Terror of Death</u>, writes, *"One can offer no greater service to someone facing death than to offer him or her your sheer presence; it is the greatest gift you can give."*

More from Yalom:

"It is the synergy between ideas and intimate connection with other people that is most effective in diminishing death anxiety... intimate relationships are a sine qua non for happiness."

In the post, "Facing Death", I mention that a very good friend of mine recently died of lymphoma. I spent time with her toward the end and I know my presence is what mattered most to her. We reminisced a lot, laughing over the many wonderful memories of our times spent together. She also liked to be reminded about all the ways she had made a difference in people's lives; she was happy that she had made "ripples" of influence. And I told her what Yalom says is the truly effective message to give to a dying friend: *"I have taken some part of you into me; it has changed and enriched me, and I will pass it on to others."*

There are some things **not** to say to someone who is sick or dying: *"It must be nice to be able to take some time off from work"* or *"Things happen for a reason"* or *"I'll pray for you"* or *"Stay strong."* These comments, besides being clichés, feel uncaring and dismissive.

I recently said something I shouldn't have to someone who is grieving the loss of his wife. I told him what stage I thought he was experiencing in his grieving process (from the stages of loss and grief described by Elizabeth Kubler-Ross in her well-known book, <u>On Death and Dying</u>). I could immediately tell that this comment was not helpful! He was obviously irritated by what I said. No one likes to be put in a generalized box. Each person's grief, whether from a terminal diagnosis or from dealing with death, is unique and personal; our conversation with them needs to be unique and personal too.

We all mean well with our words, and when someone tells me I look great I know they are just trying to be supportive. I appreciate that! And I would rather have them say that than nothing at all. But there is a better way to show support. Hopefully I've helped address this concern a bit.

Managing Stress

Recently I've written a lot about nutrition and its importance in the healing process, but reducing stress may actually play a greater role in our health. Bernie Siegel, MD, has written a lot about the impact of stress on our health (read <u>Love, Medicine, and Miracles</u>). He even says we can think ourselves sick! Studies show that excessive stress increases *cortisol* levels in our bodies, which can cause hypertension, headaches, anxiety, depression – even cancer!

While I hope that I didn't get cancer because of my thoughts, I've noticed that stress does impact me in both physiologic and psychological ways.

If stress affects our health, I need to be as stress-free as possible; those of us with cancer especially need to take good care of ourselves in this area.

I am doing my best to live a stress-free life, but stress is unavoidable. Besides the stress of cancer, I also have the inevitable conflicts with family and friends, along with all the other stressors of daily life. It seems that often the very things/people that give us the greatest joy (eustress) can also cause us the greatest stress. So I focus on spending joyful, stress-free times with my mother, my son, daughter-in-law, and three grandchildren while visiting them in California: evoking eustress! While there I also find time to have fun with my favorite cousins and old friends. When I'm with them I feel renewed and rejuvenated, appreciated, supported, and loved. They are the antidote to the negative impact of the other stressors; they help me de-stress.

Having fun is another way to de-stress and I do know how to have fun! When I was in La Jolla recently I went paragliding.

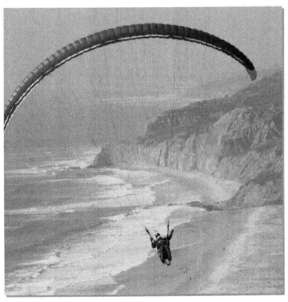

Para-Gliding in California

I went Zydeco dancing at the yearly dance festival in San Diego, Gator-by-the-Bay. I walked to my favorite beach, Windansea, in La Jolla; I walked and talked in the magnificent Redwood forest near Orinda with my son and daughter-in-law; and I enjoyed watching my grandchildren play lacrosse and tennis and soccer.

At home I've created a wonderful stress-free life for myself. I'm doing my best to take good care of my health, eating well, exercising, and reducing stress (see "Self Healing"). I live in a beautiful city, right on the water surrounded by loving, supportive friends. Every day I look out at the ducks and birds, sailboats and sunsets, and sometimes seals. I go sailing and kayaking and dancing; I watch a lot of movies and read a lot of books. I try to live each day to the fullest, as we all should.

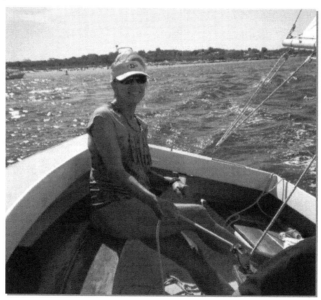

On My Sailboat

But I think it's worth considering Dr. Siegel's comment about the power of our thoughts. Much of our stress can be reduced or avoided if we just think about it differently, reframing our perspective. I'm trying to apply this new thinking to my mother's behaviors so that I will feel less stressed when I visit her. After all, according to Charles Swindoll, it's all about attitude:

The longer you live, the more you'll realize the impact of attitude on life.

Attitude is more important than the past, than education, than money, than circumstance, than failures, than successes, than what other people think or say or do.

It is more important than appearance, giftedness, or skill.

It will "make or break" a company, a church, a home.

The remarkable thing is that we all have a choice every day regarding the attitude we will embrace for that day.

We can't change our past.

We cannot change the fact that people will act in a certain way.

We cannot change the inevitable.

The only thing we can do is play on the one string we have, and that is our attitude.

This is true: life is 10% what happens to you and 90% how you react to it. And so it can be, with you...

You are in charge of your attitude!

The Benefits of Denial

Elizabeth Kubler-Ross, author of the well-known book, <u>On Death and Dying</u>, identified five stages for dealing with death; these stages have also come to be known as the five stages of grieving:

1 - Denial
2 - Anger
3 - Bargaining
4 - Depression
5 - Acceptance

I certainly have gone through each of these stages many times since getting my cancer diagnosis, but it's the *Denial Stage* I find to be the most helpful. Living with cancer "successfully" (if there is such a thing) means living with denial. Denial is *"pretending that an uncomfortable thing did not happen."* It is one of the most common defense mechanisms used; it's needed to help one continue to go on living life.

For the most part, I can pretend that I don't have Stage IV metastatic lung cancer because I am living a relatively healthy and normal life. I'm able to do just about anything I want to do. I don't look sick; I don't feel sick; people don't think I have cancer. I have learned to manage the many side effects (see "Managing Medication Side Effects") of the chemo pill Tarceva® I take daily, so that they don't interfere with my daily activities. Denial makes it possible for me to tolerate all that I'm going through; I can pretend that I'm healthy and cancer-free most of the time. It's a very helpful defense mechanism. Why not use it?

Some strategies I use for denial include dancing (see "Why I Love Zydeco Dancing"); distraction: going to movies, reading a good book, dinner with friends, exercise (walking, skiing, kayaking, practicing yoga), also long phone calls with loved ones, playing word games with friends, sailing with friends, traveling, taking care of someone else (my mother), writing in my blog, working professionally (sometimes), being outside in the sun, petting the neighbor's dog, listening to music, getting a massage, meditating, cooking nutritious meals, and much more (see "Healing Myself"). I know how to distract myself. I know how to *be in the flow*; I know how to have fun. I know how to pretend all is okay… denial.

If I didn't live in denial I would be living with fear: fear of death and dying sooner than I want; fear of experiencing painful, uncomfortable treatments to prolong my life; fear of missing out on watching my grandchildren grown up; fear of the unknown, and more.

I especially fear not leaving enough of a legacy. I want to feel that it mattered that I was here on earth – that I did something of value – that I left some sort of positive imprint on the people whose lives I've touched. The following quote from a recent newspaper article says it well: *"Every one of us, ordinary or grand, is defined by our own moments in time – by the choices we make, the obstacles we surmount, the dreams we achieve, the people we love… Whether in victory or defeat, how we choose to handle those moments is what marks the best of us long after we are gone. It is, in the end, how we are remembered."*

I want to be remembered well.

And why choose to focus on fear anyway? I deny fear! I deny anger! I deny depression! The one thing I have control over is my attitude (see "It's All About Attitude"). Therefore, I can choose to focus on the richness of my life – my special relationships, my lovely environment, my ability to play and have fun, to travel, to work, and to write. I choose to focus on doing things that matter and on fostering loving relationships with my friends and family.

There are roadblocks I run into all the time; I bump into them and then I find ways to go around them (denial?). For instance, I read blogs written by other lung cancer survivors that can be upsetting: one woman has just died after a three-year struggle; another is struggling with debilitating treatments; another is living in hospice care with limited options. I tell myself: that is *them*, this is *me*; my path will be different. But then I read in the recent CURE magazine, *"…despite positive developments (for cancer treatment) most drugs available for advanced cancer simply delay the time before the patient runs out of options… all patients build up a resistance to the drug eventually… people just aren't getting cured…."* Hard to deny. This is where I must find acceptance for my situation; I know I will run out of options sooner than later. In the meantime, denial and acceptance are my helpful coping mechanisms.

Tarceva® (my "magic bullet" chemo pill) has surely bought me some time. The average patient on Tarceva® is resistant between 14 and 20 months; I've been on the pill for more than 36 months. I seem to be the Tarceva® poster child. I try not to focus on the fear that my time is running out. I tell myself, "it's a new ball game with cancer treatments, and I will defy the odds." Others have done it; I can do it! So far, so good. I have defied the odds. But with each cat scan/MRI, denial doesn't quite overcome my anxiety until I get another "NED" (No Evidence of Disease).

Actually most of us are in denial about our deaths. Before Cancer (B.C.) I was like you: thinking that death was a long way off. I planned to live into my 90's (like my mother). Unfortunately, a cancer diagnosis puts death in one's face; then it's hard to deny. All of a sudden my best plan is to live into my 70's.

However, it's important to not always be in denial; it is important to face death sometimes. It's helpful at times to remember that we are all going to die and that we never know when. If we remember, then we are more likely to value the present moment. We become more mindful and, hopefully, live each day as if it were our last; this makes each day special. Our priorities become clearer and we make better choices.

I'm very aware of the value of each day. I'm very aware of what matters most to me (my relationships). I'm certainly aware that death is closer, but denial helps me live each day to the fullest. I guess there needs to be some balance between denial and accepting the reality of death (see "The Black Box"). I also know I need to acknowledge and express my feelings of anger and depression at times (the other stages).

Being hopeful and optimistic and accepting is so much more pleasant than being fearful or angry or depressed. Denial makes that possible. I plan to *be in denial* for a very long time as I'm *Dancing Through Cancer*.

Unexpected Risks

Ideally we want to choose the risks we take, but sometimes we are thrown into a situation that forces us to take risks we haven't chosen – getting a cancer diagnosis does just that! It is unexpected, unwelcome, and disorienting, yet we must learn to cope as best we can. The dictionary defines risk as "exposure to harm, peril, hazard, or loss." My cancer diagnosis was certainly an unexpected risk.

One day I was living in the **comfort zone** of my life, the next day I was pushed over the edge into a new zone: the panic zone. The **panic zone** is not where any of us wants to be. It's a zone filled with fear, anxiety, uncertainty, confusion, depression, anger; all of which can be overwhelming. Eventually we are forced to face these feelings and muster the courage to deal with our new situation. We can then move out of the panic zone into a new zone where we learn new strategies to deal with the consequences of the risk we have been forced to take; this is the **learning zone**. The learning zone is an unknown area where we figure out how to live a **"new normal life"** that becomes our **"new comfort zone."**

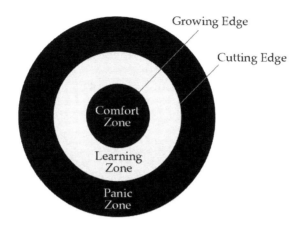

When I got my lung cancer diagnosis, the unexpected risk, I was in shock and disbelief. I felt like I'd just jumped off the edge of a tall building, free-falling into the unknown. I certainly felt panic; I didn't know how to deal with all the emotions welling up within me. Slowly I gained control of my life – I got wings! - and, little by little, with a lot of help from my friends and family and physicians, I have learned how to live in my new comfort zone.

I have learned a lot over the years (nearly five and counting). I have done my best to educate myself about lung cancer and all the treatment options available: those recommended by western medicine physicians, integrative physicians, experts in alternative treatments (acupuncture, acupressure, meditation, yoga, Reiki, Tong Ren therapy...), nutritionists, and other cancer patients. I have learned, and continue to learn, ways to live with lung cancer. I've been *Dancing Through Cancer*, enjoying life as best I can. My blog documents all my learning; it has been a means for me to clarify what has been helpful, as well as a means to educate others on ways to prevent and, hopefully, heal from cancer.

I've written a lot in the past about risk-taking (see my website www.ingearcoaching.com, also my book "Risk to Grow! Create the Life You Want Through Responsible Risk-Taking"). There I explain how best to choose risks we want to take in order to grow. Taking risks always forces us to grow, whether we choose them or not. I didn't choose to get cancer, but I know I have grown immensely from this unexpected risk. Most important, I have learned what matters most to me: my relationships with my family and friends. I have also learned how to eat much more healthfully. I have learned how to reduce my stress and enjoy life. I have learned how to meditate and to live more mindfully. I have learned to be grateful for each day and grateful for all the richness in my life.

My friends tell me that I am a different person; they frequently remark on my positive attitude and my courage while dealing with cancer. I didn't know that I would become this person, but I am pleased that I have grown in such a way. Getting cancer certainly forced me to take many unexpected risks, and I do think I am a better person for it.

What risks, unexpected or planned, have you taken in your life? How have you grown? What have you learned? What risks can you plan to take that will help you grow? How can you best prepare for any unexpected risks?

No one can predict a cancer diagnosis or any other unexpected risk, but you can do your best to develop healthful practices and strategies to be prepared, just in case.

The Spirit of Hope Award

I just received the "Spirit of Hope" award from the International Coach Federation of New England (viewed at www.icfne.org). This award is given to the coach who demonstrates a strong spirit in the face of challenging odds. I was the first recipient.

I wasn't able to attend the ceremony so I sent these words to be read by a fellow coach:

Dear ICFNE membership,

I am very touched by this honor and sorry that I am not able to be here tonight to accept the award in person; I had a previous commitment.

Although I really don't think I deserve this award since it doesn't seem to me that I'm doing anything differently from what any one of you would do if you had my cancer diagnosis. We all just manage the best we can with what we're given in life.

It helps that I feel well and have lots of energy. I'm not sure my attitude would be so positive if I were tired or nauseous or in pain.

Getting an unexpected diagnosis like this has a way of having us prioritize our life's goals in an instant. I immediately knew that what is most important to me is being with my family and friends – not work, not travel – so now I spend as much time as possible with the people I love. It's especially important to me to make memories with my grandchildren.

I couldn't go through this difficult journey without my friends – and many of you are among them. I appreciate so much all your encouraging comments on my Carepages; all this support means so much to me!

Lung cancer is the single biggest killer of cancers, so it's not a great diagnosis to get, especially for a non-smoker. However, with all the new research and treatment options, I am optimistic that I will be one of the growing number of people living with cancer for a very long while.

I'm glad if I can be an inspiration of spirit and hope to other people touched by cancer. For this reason I am writing a new blog, "Dancing Through Cancer," which you can access at www.ingearcoaching.com/blog (also through Facbook or Twitter).

Our society focuses almost completely on the treatment of cancer rather than on the prevention of cancer. So the coach in me encourages you to do your best to educate yourself on the most effective ways to prevent cancer from becoming a disease you have to deal with!

Again… thank you all for honoring me with this very special award; I will always cherish it.

Sincerely, Laurie

My Support System

A Little Help From My Friends

When I got my lung cancer diagnosis I immediately realized that what matters most to me is being with my family and friends. Cancer has a way of immediately focusing our attention on what and whom we care about most. My bucket list no longer seemed important. I had one desire: to spend as much time as possible, for as long as I can, with the people I love.

Traveling to many exotic places had been on my bucket list. However, I know that on my death bed I won't be thinking about all the places I've been; I'll be remembering and relishing all my relationships. If, on the other hand, I can travel with friends (or family) and share adventures with them, then that will be the best scenario. And that's what I just did.

I recently spent over two weeks with three amazing women friends (and visiting two other amazing women friends) in France (the Pyrenees) and Spain (Cadaques, Barcelona, Madrid). It was an unforgettable trip: we laughed and cried and celebrated together as we hiked and biked and explored and shopped, ate and drank. There's nothing like the special intimacy and connection that can happen when women are together. We created many wonderful memories that I will always cherish.

I've done a lot of reading and writing on affiliations (see my website: www.ingearcoaching.com) and it's interesting that many research studies report that social contact is found to be the single most important factor in longevity. Also, that isolated people were found to have a death rate two to four times higher than others.

Dr. Edward Hallowell, in his book, <u>Connect</u>, says, "*To thrive, indeed just to survive, we need warmhearted contact with other people... Like a vitamin deficiency, human contact deficiency weakens the body, the mind, the spirit.*" According to him we need a daily dose of Vitamin C (C=Connection!).

I certainly get my daily dose of Vitamin "C". I feel so supported and nurtured and affirmed and appreciated by my friends; I live in a cocoon of caring and loving kindness. I couldn't go through this cancer journey without them. They've been here for me all along the way: in the hospital, in the infusion room, at the doctor's office, during procedures, in my home and theirs. I am grateful each and every day for their love and support.

Another study on aging showed that one of the most powerful predictors of well being in old age is the frequency of visits with friends. I'm sure the frequency of visits with friends prolongs life, too. And when we're gone it's those memories (like our wonderful trip) that keep us alive in other people's lives.

This African love poem also says it well:

"A friend is someone who knows your song and sings it to you when you have forgotten it.

Those who love you are not fooled by mistakes you have made or dark images you hold about yourself.

They remember your beauty when you feel ugly; your wholeness when you are broken; your innocence when you feel guilty; and your purpose when you are confused."

Maya Angelou said, *"I've learned that people will forget what you said, people will forget what you did, but people will never forget how you made them feel."*

My other goal is to make my friends feel as cherished and nourished as I feel from them. So...
I try with a little help from my friends
I get high with a little help from my friends
I get by with a little help from my friends...
~ written by Ringo with the Beatles
(See "Acknowledgments" to read about my complete support network.)

My Women's Group

We've been meeting for almost 20 years. There were eight of us initially; we formed a group in order to explore what spirituality meant to us. We were Catholics, Jews, Christians, and an Agnostic. We hired two other women friends in Divinity School to guide us in our discussions for a six-week course. Six of us decided to continue to meet over the years; our two leaders left once they finished their programs, and the other two women decided that the bi-weekly commitment was too much.

We meet every other week. Two of us take turns facilitating; we generally focus on a topic. We light candles, burn sage, read poetry, meditate – all to help us be in the present moment and shed extraneous distractions.

Besides spirituality, we discuss many other life issues: dealing with aging parents, dealing with our own aging, parenting, relationships, health concerns, planning for the future, professional and personal life transitions, etc. We celebrate together at weddings and births and major birthday milestones; we've supported each other through deaths and divorce and disease. We have also gone on trips together, attended workshops and concerts and plays together, and we regularly get together for coffee. We have a lot of fun whenever we are together. We are the kind of family each of us would choose to have: the most loving and caring family one could ever imagine.

And these women have been completely loving and caring of me during my cancer journey. They visited me in the hospital, they took turns going with me to doctor appointments and procedures, they took care of me in their homes after chemotherapy infusions, they created a healing circle for me, they made me meals, they call to check in on me regularly. I know they will be here whenever I need them. I imagine them surrounding me with loving kindness on my deathbed, easing my passing.

I feel so grateful and blessed.

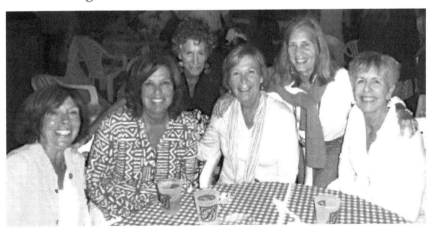

My Women's Group

Life Lessons from Babies

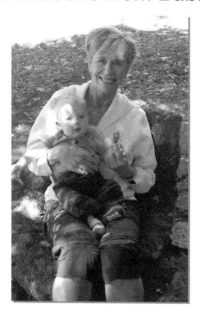

My Great Nephew, Felix

We should all see the world through the eyes of a baby! I just spent a couple of weeks with my great nephew, Felix (age 10 months in 2011), and was fascinated by the way he sees the world. I realized I could learn a lot from him. I was reminded of all I have forgotten about how to live life fully.

Felix pops up in his bed each morning with big bright eyes and a smile on his face, eager to start his day. Each day brings new discoveries and new skills. It's wonderful to see his fascination with anything new and different, and he gets so excited when he manages to master some new skill. Falling down or making mistakes are only bumps in the road; he just gets right back up and starts over with renewed determination. He takes risks and overcomes challenges with ease.

I want to wake up each day and look forward to all the possibilities a new day will bring. I want to keep learning and growing. I don't want to let mistakes or failings deter me. I want to take more risks. I want to play more and have more fun.

And, like Felix, I want to laugh a lot. There's nothing like his laugh! When I'm around him I find myself smiling and laughing all the time. He makes me feel joyful and happy because he is so delighted with all he is experiencing. I smile as I write this just thinking about him.

Felix also shows me how to live in the moment; the present is all he knows. When he's interested in something, he completely focuses on it and gives it his total attention.

I can learn from this!

Felix expresses his feelings in the moment too; we know immediately when he's mad or sad or happy or afraid. He lets us know just how he feels and what he wants; nothing is ambiguous or unclear. And he gives his love unconditionally.

Felix shows me what it means to live a fulfilling life; I want to live just like this.

Life lessons to be learned from Felix (and other babies):

- be present; live in the moment
- give unconditional love
- laugh a lot
- be playful - as much as you can
- express all your feelings, both good and bad
- learn from mistakes - be determined
- never stop learning new things and new skills
- take risks
- grow and change
- love life and have fun!

Thank you, Felix, for teaching me how to live life to the fullest!

Sick and Single

I was alone when I got the news that I had lung cancer. I'll never forget that moment – like how none of us will ever forget when we heard that JFK was shot or when the twin towers were hit. My diagnosis was totally unexpected (never having been a smoker). I had gone in for a routine chest x-ray in preparation for a breast lumpectomy (see "My Story"). As soon as I got home I received the call from my breast surgeon: "I'm sorry to tell you that you have lung cancer." I remember standing there with the phone in my hand in utter disbelief, shaking, having my first out-of-body experience.

What I needed and wanted right then was for someone to hold me and comfort me. But there was no one there. So I immediately got on the phone and began calling my friends and family; I needed to feel connected. They were there for me virtually, for which I am so grateful! But it's not the same as being there for me in person. I lived alone and far away from any of them.

After that, everyone rallied around me. People took turns accompanying me to doctor appointments, medical procedures, surgery, hospital stays, and chemotherapy infusions. My friends took turns taking care of me in their homes on "recovery" weekends after chemo; my younger son came up from New York to care for me; my older son and family took me into their home and cared for me for two months post lung surgery. I felt loved and supported; I was well cared for. Now, living with cancer and with the on-going side effects from the chemo pill I must take daily, my friends and family continue to be there for me.

Despite all this amazing support, I am alone a lot; often when I need a hug there's no one here. I know I could call someone to come over, but that doesn't solve the immediate need. It's usually in the middle of the night when I feel alone. Thus I sometimes find myself envying the cancer survivors who have a life partner who will hug and hold them whenever they want, especially in the wee hours of the night. It can be lonely late at night facing my fears and feeling discomfort; I often just want to get into a fetal position and be held. Being single means being alone at times when you don't want to be alone.

However, I look at the many positives of being single. Because I'm single my friends are more attentive and supportive; they are much more willing to do whatever I ask for whenever I need it. My sons are more loving and make more of an effort to care for me. In fact, my younger son has moved back to Gloucester in order to be closer to me; this is such a gift of loving care. I cherish our times together.

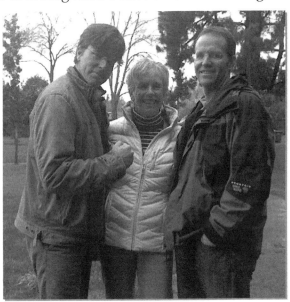

With My Sons, Derek and Scott

A good friend, Francine, who happens to be a nurse, has designated herself as my personal health care advocate and goes with me to every oncology appointment. She drives down from Vermont (four hours away) to support me. Other friends go with me to my MRI appointments or other medical procedures as needed. And then there's my women's group (see "My Women's Group") who support me in every way they can; they are like an extended family. I know I can call on them whenever I need help.

One reason I chose to move back to Gloucester was so that I would be close enough to my friends. I feel that my relationships have been enriched and enhanced by my lung cancer experience; I feel closer to everyone. I experience loving kindness at every turn. I don't think I would be getting this kind of support if I weren't single. This is the "Single Silver Lining."

The richness of my connections cannot be measured. Because I'm single I am held in a different way – perhaps a more powerful and supportive way – than just being held by one person. And I know my friends would even hold me tightly in the middle of the night if I called on them to come over.

I may be sick and single, but I'm not alone at all, and I know I never will be.

Spirituality

My Spiritual Journey

I had no religious or spiritual education growing up. I never went to church unless a friend wanted me to accompany her after a sleepover. My mother called herself an *atheist*. I wasn't sure what I believed, so I called myself an *agnostic*.

I was exposed to religion nevertheless, but my experiences were all pretty negative. I attended an Episcopalian school for 7th and 8th grades (The Bishop's School in La Jolla, CA). We had to go to chapel two mornings a week. I hated going because we had to stand for long periods of time singing psalms and saying prayers. Girls would frequently faint and be carried out; I always worried I would be one of them. Thankfully, my mother gave me smelling salts, which seemed to work (since I never fainted). We also had to spend an inordinate amount of time (it seemed) memorizing and reciting psalms during the week. I just didn't see the point in all that.

When I was 14 my mother moved us to Torremolinos, Spain. The only school nearby was a Catholic Convent in Malaga: "Colegio de la Asuncion." My sister and I lived separately in the dormitory, so this was total immersion – complete culture shock! We had to attend Mass every morning and all day on Holy Days (there are a *lot* of Holy Days in Spain!). Of course this was all delivered in Latin and Spanish. The experience was confusing, meaningless, and just plain boring. Fortunately we were only there for about six months (read more about my experience in "Gidget Goes to the Convent").

When married we never attended church as a family; sports events always seemed to take precedence. (Years later, my older son complained that he had been deprived by never getting a religious education; I tell him it's never too late!)

My father was a devoted Episcopalian, never missing a Sunday in church. Whenever I visited him I would accompany him. However, I was turned off by the minister, hearing him say, *"We are the one true church."* I found the service to be exclusive and sexist (every pronoun was "he").

So, what does spirituality mean to me? That's the key question I've been trying to answer for years.

I think spirituality means believing in a greater good… a higher power… believing in something greater than ourselves, and believing that we are all connected somehow to this greater energy/force that also comes from within us. Spirituality is an inner state of peace or grace. Spirituality lacks a clear definition for everyone, it seems; there are actually over 500 definitions of spirituality on the Internet. Spirituality means something different to each person; one's spirituality is very personal. I think we each have to find our own definition. I think I've found mine, finally.

I found my definition of spirituality after one woman in our women's group led me to Buddhism. She has been involved in a local Buddhist center that has grown over the years, offering many teachings and practices. I attended many of the public talks given by the Lama Marut, an American Buddhist monk (visit www.lamamarut.org), and always found his teachings of the Buddhist principles to be very compelling and relevant. The principles come closest to defining for me what spirituality means (see "Principles of Buddhism"). Finally, I seem to have found a spiritual path that makes sense to me!

Buddhism seems to be inclusive and practical; there's no dogma. I felt moved to explore more so I decided to attend the summer retreat (see next post), which has certainly helped me to understand and experience more of the principles. The more I learn the more I am moved to follow this spiritual path. It has taken over 60 years, but I've finally found a way to live a more spiritual life. I know my newfound spirituality will help me live more peacefully while managing cancer, and I have faith that I will be at peace on my deathbed.

Buddhist Summer Retreat

I've never had much of a spiritual life, but now that I have lung cancer, it seems important to develop one. A local Buddhist center holds a yearly summer retreat, so I decided I wanted to attend this year (2012). There were over 100 of us from all over the U.S. and Canada. For six days we listened to teachings by four different spiritual guides: Lama Marut, Cindy Lee, Lindsay Crouse, and her husband, Rick Blue. We meditated and practiced yoga daily, and we went into silence for two-and-a-half days (no talking, no email, no phones). This experience has had a profound, life-changing affect on me.

There are many changes I now plan to make in my life. I am committed to meditate every day, even if only for five minutes; I plan to write in a gratitude journal daily; I plan to practice yoga at least twice a week; mostly I plan to live the teachings of the Buddhist principles as best I can. I want to create good karma for my future, however limited it might be.

Buddhism has a strong spiritual history and tradition; its teachings have survived for over 2500 years. Other religious traditions – Christianity, Judaism, and Hinduism – have embraced the same basic teaching: *"Do unto others as you would have others do unto you"* (that's karma). What attracts me most to Buddhism is its main goal in life: *to be happy* (and the best way to be happy is to make someone else happy). In the next post I will write about all the other principles that can help one to lead a happy life. For now, I'm off to meditate.

Principles of Buddhism

The principles of Buddhism center around the basic goal of living a happy life. What could be better than that? Here are many of the principles that attract me – principles that I want to live by:

- Happiness: Life is all about happiness. The main purpose in life is to be happy, yet, according to Lama Marut, many people have euphobia: the fear of being happy. Living the principles of Buddhism is the path to happiness, but it takes time. Lama Marut recommends that you fake happiness until you get happy; "fake it 'til you make it" (and then you will!). Many of these Buddhist principles show us all the ways to be happy. "The purpose of our lives is to be happy." H.H. the 14th Dalai Lama

- Karma: Karma is the result of a previous action, a cause, which leads to a result. Everything is caused; therefore, I want to do my best to create good results – good karma. What goes around comes around. This means making others happy, giving service, being compassionate, offering loving-kindness and random acts of kindness, being generous, grateful, and patient, finding forgiveness, living an ethical and moral life.

• Mindfulness: Mindfulness means living completely in the present moment, to be here now. I want to stop being so distracted and scattered, reduce multi-tasking and addictive behaviors (email, texting, movies), stop the mind-chatter and negative self-talk. I want to be more present to my friends and family, my colleagues and clients. The present is actually all we have, so why not enjoy it? (see "The Best Present is Presence (At Christmas)"). Meditation is the best method I know to help me learn to be more mindful (see "Committing to Meditation").

• Subjectivity: Our world is viewed through our own subjective filters; everything is filtered through our perceptions, which were created by our past experiences and our relationships. Therefore, we can always change our view of things if we don't like what's happening; there's always another way of looking at the situation. We can't change the present, but we can change our reaction to what's happening in the present. We can actually change the past by choosing what we focus on in our memories (we do it all the time, really). So do we want to focus on the positive parts of the memory or on the negative parts? Which would make us happier? The same goes for the future. Do we want to focus on things that will make us feel anxious and fearful or do we want to focus on things that will make us feel excited and hopeful? We can choose; it's all subjective. I choose happiness.

- <u>Death</u>: Buddhism acknowledges, even embraces death. Most of us live with a somewhat magical belief that death won't happen to us, or at least we think it is a long way off. Not so for those of us given a cancer diagnosis; and not so for many others with an illness! Buddhism focuses on two key points about death: 1) Death is certain; we are all going to die. 2) We never know when we will die. Therefore we need to think about what actions we can take now in order to live a full and happy life. Lama Marut recommends that we focus on these key points each morning, saying to ourself: "If today were my last day on earth, how will I live it?" That day is bound to be very special. (For more thoughts on death, read "Facing Death").

- <u>Contentment</u>: To be content I acknowledge that my life is fine just the way it is; I have enough! I need only think about all that I have and be grateful every day. I accept that life is – and that I am – perfect.

- <u>Take Responsibility</u>: I need to take responsibility for my own actions and not blame others. I am in charge of my own reactions.

- <u>Be Disciplined</u>: I need to be disciplined in my practice of the Buddhist principles.

- <u>Change</u>: Change is another certainty in life; everything is always changing. So if you're feeling sad or anxious or irritated, you can be comforted knowing that these feelings will change. On the other hand, if you're feeling happy or excited or loving, these feelings will change too. Just remembering that things will always change brings me a certain peace of mind.

- <u>Interdependence</u>: We are all interdependent; we interact in relation to everyone else. We are like waves in an ocean: the waves are part of the whole ocean and each wave affects the others. Therefore, we need to care for others as we care for ourselves: do unto others as you would have others do unto you. We need to learn to embrace our commonality and our ordinariness. Ironically, the messages of the "American Dream" are to be just the opposite: "Be Extraordinary - Be All You Can Be - Be a Maverick - Go for the Gold." These messages are all designed for us to become independent and to feel unique and special, but they also separate us into winners and losers. The few who "make it" may achieve fleeting happiness, but the many who don't measure up are not very happy.

- <u>Attachment</u>: Our desire for things (computers, iPads, iPhones, cars, clothes, jewelry, trips, etc.) keeps us in a constant state of dissatisfaction; there's always something more we need to buy. We may achieve fleeting happiness with the newest thing, but we so quickly lose that happiness. The problem is that we are "looking for happiness in all the wrong places" (according to Lama Marut). We keep looking externally: we want a better house, a better car, a better job, a better relationship, the next vacation, more money, and so on. But lasting happiness is actually found within us; we need to look internally. The Buddhist principles guide us to find happiness within.

- <u>Our Greatest Teachers</u>: These are the people who cause us the most problems - our most irritating, toxic people; through them we learn humility, compassion, patience, and how to find love in the face of conflict.

These principles are what attracted me to Buddhism. I want to live as happy a life as possible in all the time I have left. I know I am going to die and it may be sooner than I want, but I know if I can live these principles I will live a happier life now.

Lama Marut's new book, <u>A Spiritual Renegade's Guide to the Good Life</u>, gives a much clearer description of all the Buddhist principles I've mentioned and much more. I highly recommend reading it.

Committing to Meditation

I recently attended a week-long meditation retreat with Jack Kornfield at the Kripalu Center for Yoga and Health. I had gone thinking I would learn more about Buddhist principles, which I have been attracted to for the past few years; I learned much more than I thought possible.

Kornfield, an American trained as a Buddhist monk, is one of the key teachers to introduce Buddhist practices to the West (he has written many books). He seems to be a truly spiritual being; he just radiates love and compassion. When I spoke to him I felt his total presence and connection with me. Being around him and watching the way he interacted with everyone else was what mainly motivated me to embrace his teachings. I'd like to be more like him.

There were almost 200 of us at the retreat, people from all over the U.S. (he's very well-known and has quite the following). Jack shared his teachings, bringing them alive with moving and funny stories. And then we meditated… and meditated… and meditated.

I've never been a meditator. I've always thought it is a good practice to have, but I could never seem to find the time to sit still and focus. I am now convinced that the commitment is worth the effort. And I know I can find 15 minutes out of each day to meditate (I'll just subtract some of the time I spend on the computer!).

What I learned from Jack (and the other two speakers), from the other participants (many seasoned meditators), and from all the books I'm reading, are the many potential benefits of a meditation practice:

- Creating mindfulness; learning to be totally in the present: Be Here Now.

- Easing the mind / letting go of suffering.

- Creating more joy.

- Learning to forgive.

- Reducing patterns of unhelpful worry and obsession, destructive views and opinions.

- Becoming less judgmental.

- Clarifying confusion; making better decisions.

- Reconnecting with our heart and discovering an inner sense of spaciousness, unity, and compassion.

- Reflecting more deeply on what we value.

- Being grateful each and every day; developing an attitude of gratitude.

- Focusing on loving kindness in myself, as well as in others.

- Finding peace and happiness.

These potential benefits motivate me to commit to a daily meditation practice. Being mindful will surely help me be more present to my coaching clients and to friends and family in distress. It should help me be less distracted and forgetful. Most importantly, it will help me be more present and thus live each day to the fullest.

From Jack's book, <u>A Path with Heart:</u>

"Meditation can be thought of as the art of awakening. Through the mastering of this art we can learn new ways to approach our difficulties and bring wisdom and joy alive in our life. Through developing meditation's tools and practices we can awaken the best of our spiritual human capacities. The key to this art is the steadiness of our attention."

Meditating isn't easy. Basic meditation practice means focusing on the breath. I find it very hard to keep my focus on the breath, as my mind is constantly focusing on plans for the future, memories of the past, or other random thoughts. I'm assured that the more I practice meditating the more I will be able to stay with the breath. Like any new skill, it takes time to learn it. So my intention is to meditate daily – even if only for five minutes – for one month (they say it takes four to six weeks to create a new habit). I know that my efforts will be worth it; I trust that I will reap the benefits.

Future Planning

Getting My Teeth Whitened: Planning for the Future!

I've decided to get my teeth whitened. This may not sound like a big deal, but it really is. It means I'm planning on the future; it means I'm planning to be around long enough to enjoy whiter teeth.

I've read many stories from people with advanced cancer who say they just want to be alive long enough to see their children graduate or to see a child married or to see a grandchild being born... and they make it! This says something about the power of intention and hope. I like knowing that my attitude and determination can help me prolong my life... and enjoy it longer too.

I recently read Dan Brown's book, The Lost Symbol, where he comments on the power of intention: "*Human thought can literally transform the physical world – we are the masters of our own universe. At the subatomic level... particles themselves come in and out of existence based solely on one's intention... in a sense, one's desire to see a particle manifests that particle. Living consciousness somehow is the influence that turns the possibility of something into something real.*"

My thoughts – my attitude – can influence my outcomes. It is certainly something to ponder!

Of course it's not about my teeth. I'm holding out to see my grandchildren graduate from high school (college?) and see them married (and have children, too). It's a grand scheme and it's optimistic, but I will do all I can to believe in this possibility. I plan to have a future with my grandchildren!

Financial Planning

How can I make a financial plan for the future when I don't know how much of a future I have? This is the dilemma of everyone who has a Stage IV cancer diagnosis.

I live on social security, a small retirement fund, and occasional consulting work. My financial planner tells me that I will run out of money within eight to nine years if I continue to live my current lifestyle. Can I expect to live that long? Doubtful, according to the statistics (only 5% of people with end-stage lung cancer survive longer than 5 years). I don't want to be like my friend, Rheua, whose financial plan meant saving enough to live to be 90, but who died unexpectedly at 65 of Chronic Lymphocytic Leukemia (CLL). She sacrificed in the present so that she would have money for her future, but she never got to her future.

Cancer takes people's lives sooner than expected, thus, with a cancer diagnosis, I think one should live for *now*. My philosophy is to spend my money and enjoy life in the present, as the future may never arrive.

So I shall continue to live my lifestyle, which includes spending time with my friends and family, while traveling, dancing, skiing, sailing, integrating alternative healing modalities and self care (see "Self-Healing - Alternative Medicine"), writing in my blog (to become this book), and not working much so that I have the time to do all this. I'm glad I have this choice.

Living With the Unknown

Living with lung cancer means living with the unknown... mainly living with the fear of the unknown. I know death will be coming to me sooner than expected, but I don't know when. I do know how: complications due to lung cancer. Statistics tell me I should be dead by now, but I defy statistics as I approach the five-year mark post-diagnosis. Therefore, I am now "in unchartered territory" (as my oncologist frequently tells me).

I don't fear death. After reading numerous books about death and near-death experiences (see "Resources" and "Facing Death"), I think death will be peaceful and possibly even transformative and enlightening. What I fear are the complications and suffering I may experience leading up to death; those are the scary unknowns. I read blogs by other lung cancer survivors or hear of other experiences; it seems that everyone eventually goes through a variety of complicated, even torturous, treatments. Clinical trials, more chemotherapy infusions, more medical or surgical procedures are all part of the process of keeping people alive. I read how uncomfortable – sick, tired, nauseous, debilitated – people get, and it scares me. I worry that their path will be my path.

The western medicine approach to treating cancer is to poison the cancer cells. However, in the process, healthy cells are also poisoned (see film: "Cut, Poison, Burn" in "Resources"). The theory is that the healthy cells will out-survive the cancer cells, and this is what mostly happens. But the cancer patient can get *very sick* in the process, and sometimes the patient does not survive the treatment. When does one know that enough is enough? What if I want to "go" but my loved ones don't want me to? I suspect most people put up with the torturous treatments because they are hoping a cure will be discovered, or they want to ease the suffering of their loved ones, or they want to buy more time. But do they suffer unnecessarily? I don't want to suffer like that, yet I know it will be hard to decide to let go when I get to that stage.

Another lung cancer patient, Teri Simon (see her book: <u>Perspectives of a Flying Elephant: My First Year in the Land of Lung Junk</u>), finally gave up the fight after months of suffering painful treatments. She ultimately wrote in her blog, *"Currently, cancer treatment is doing more to destroy my healthy body than it is to kill the cancer, and this just is no way for me to live. I no longer want to live like this. I hope you will respect this choice I have made and hope with me for peaceful outcomes."* I read later that she had a beautiful and peaceful passing surrounded by all her loved ones.

I did not like to read about all the painful treatments she went through before she died, but I respect her courage in choosing to let go. Maybe I will know when to let go too, but it's certainly an unknown.

Another fear concerns the repercussions of all the chemicals and treatments that my body is being exposed to now. I've read that cat scans can cause cancer; I have a cat scan every three months! I have an MRI frequently. I had SRS (Stereotactic RadioSurgery) to the brain (and may need more SRS). I have also had poisonous chemicals coursing through my body for almost five years. No one knows how all this will affect me long term. Another unknown.

None of us knows what the future will bring. We are all going to die and we never know when; everyone lives with the unknown to a certain extent. But it's just that the unknown is a little more prevalent when one has cancer.

I know there's no point in worrying about the unknown, so I do my best to be in denial (see "The Benefits of Denial") and take the best care of myself as I can (see "Healing Myself"). I remind myself that all we have is *today*, so I do my best to enjoy each day and focus on what's good in my life. I continue to *Dance Through Cancer!*

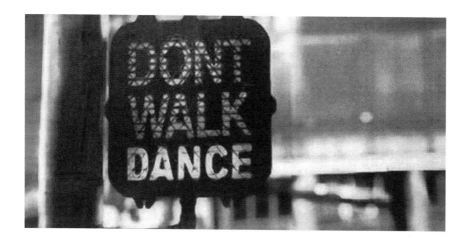

Death & Dying

Facing Death

I've recently had an "awakening experience." According to Irvin Yalom in his remarkable book: <u>Staring at the Sun: Overcoming the Fear of Death</u>, an "awakening experience" is a trigger event that causes you to face your own mortality. Getting diagnosed with cancer is clearly an awakening experience. But my recent awakening experience was the death of a very dear friend of mine (due to complications with leukemia). And just last March I had another one when the husband of another good friend died unexpectedly of a stroke.

"Awakening" triggers can be big birthdays (turning 50-60-70-80…), major life milestones (weddings, anniversaries, reunions), retirement, job loss, empty nest, cataclysmic trauma (a robbery or a car accident, etc.), and even dreams. We face these events throughout our lifetime; our existence is forever shadowed by the knowledge that we will inevitably diminish and die. But this is not a bad thing. According to Yalom, the idea of death saves us because confronting death has the potential to motivate us to live a more enriching, compassionate, and *fulfilling life.*

St. Augustine (of the Third century) once said *"It is only in the face of death that a man's self is born."*

Death is our destiny, yet most of us (me included, BC: Before Cancer) try not to think about death. It seems to be such a long way off that we live as if it isn't going to happen to us. This is *Magical Thinking*!

An awakening experience puts death in our face once again, but how quickly we forget.

What's the problem with forgetting? We think (falsely) that we have all the time in the world, so we may put up with things that bother us, or put off doing things that are important to us. Instead we ought to take advantage of our awakening experiences to ask ourselves:

- Am I living the life I want?

- Am I happy?

- Am I surrounded by people who nourish me?

- Do I have meaning and purpose in my life?

- Am I "giving back"?

- Am I making a difference?

- When I look back at my life on my deathbed, will I feel I have lived a happy, meaningful life?

- What do I regret? Can I forgive myself for my regrets? How can I live my life so I don't accumulate more regrets?

I think the more regrets we have, the harder it will be to face death. There's nothing we can do about the past, except forgive ourselves for actions we regret, but we do have control over our present and future. The value of regret is that it can be a tool to help us take actions to prevent further regret.

My friend was worried that she would be forgotten when she died, especially since she had never had children. I assured her that she had made a difference in many people's lives; the memory of her would always be there. Someone once said, "Look for her among her friends." I know I will always see her in her many friends and colleagues; and I told her that a part of her is within me, too.

Yalom said that the truly effective message to give a dying friend is *"...that I have taken some part of you into me; it has changed and enriched me, and I will pass it on to others."*

I also found these words from Sue Miller (<u>When She Was Gone</u>) to be very comforting: *"...memory itself is a living metaphor for the eternal life. Loss brings pain... but pain triggers memory... memory can change pain into laughter, to joy... to bring the dead back into our lives..."*

It has been said somewhere that there are two deaths when someone dies: (1) the actual, physical death (2) the final death when people stop talking about the deceased.

Mexicans don't forget their loved ones. *El Dia de los Muertos* (the Mexican *Day of the Dead*) is celebrated every year in order to keep the memory of their dead loved ones alive. Traditions vary from region to region, but generally families gather at cemeteries to tend and decorate the graves of their departed loved ones and remember them by telling stories, eating their favorite foods, and dancing in their honor. Many families build altars at home, decorated with flowers and food, especially *pan de muerto* or *bread of the dead*. A festive and social occasion, the holiday welcomes the return of those who have died and recognizes the human cycle of life and death.

When a Jewish person dies, their family says Kaddish every day for a month, then once a week for the rest of the year, then once a year for as long as a member of the family lives. I love these traditions. I hope I am remembered in some of these ways!

Eckhart Tolle, in his remarkable book, <u>A New Earth</u>, has another point of view on life and death that I find fascinating. He states that the human body is made up of *form* and *formless*. Form is our physical body with all its solid parts: our organs, blood vessels, muscles, etc. Formless is all the inner space in between the Form. Our physical body is actually 99.9% empty space, which, according to Tolle is a microcosmic version of the vastness of outer space. Some call this inner space "chi" or "energy" or "soul"; Tolle sees our inner space as life in its fullness. I see it as our basic essence – who we are.

So when we die, our Form dissolves, but where does our Formless go? I imagine it goes out into the universe and joins all the other "Formless spaces" of people who have passed away. So, like memory, we never really leave. Life eternal?

Buddhists believe that we pass on to another life by becoming reincarnated; our Formlessness passes on into another Form.

I take comfort in all this... How about you?

Another concept Yalom describes is one of "rippling": *"Rippling refers to the fact that each of us creates – often without our conscious intent or knowledge – concentric circles of influence that may affect others for years, even generations... Rippling refers to leaving behind something from your life experience, some trait, some piece of wisdom, guidance, virtue, or comfort that passes on to others, known or unknown."*

Knowing that once I die I will be remembered through my actions and experiences and teachings, which may ripple through generations to come, is a powerful consolation in facing a death that may come earlier than expected. And, like my friend, I'd like to be a role model of how to die gracefully and peacefully, with courage and dignity, leaving lots of ripples. I also like to think that my blogs and this book will have ripple effects.

Another recent book, <u>Proof of Heaven: A Neurosurgeon's Journey into the Afterlife</u>, by Eben Alexander, MD, has had a big impact on me. He is a scientist/physician who had a very convincing NDE (Near Death Experience), which he describes scientifically and medically. His story has been called "remarkable and revolutionary"; it's certainly compelling and convincing! Based on his personal experience, he strongly believes that death is not the end of existence, but only a transition; he is convinced that there is an afterlife. I find this very comforting. During his NDE the main message that he received was that the true meaning of life is *love* (see "Conclusion" for his words).

Those of us living with cancer stare death in the face regularly. Some people have even said cancer is a gift (although it's a gift I'd love to return!). The gift is that it helps us value what is most important to us. If I have less time on this earth, then I'm going to try to be only with people I care about and not be around people who create stress in my life. I am only going to do what I want to do and not do things I don't want to do. I will do my best to surround myself with beauty and to appreciate all the beauty around me. I'll live each day as if it were my last. I'll be grateful each and every day for being alive.

Steve Jobs died recently. A commencement speech he gave in 2005 is worth including here with the powerful comments he makes about facing his own mortality when he was diagnosed with cancer: *"When I was 17, I read a quote that went something like: 'If you live each day as if it was your last, someday you'll most certainly be right.' It made an impression on me, and since then, for the past 33 years, I have looked in the mirror every morning and asked myself, 'If today were the last day of my life, would I want to do what I am about to do today?' And whenever the answer has been 'No' for too many days in a row, I know I need to change something.*

Remembering that I'll be dead soon is the most important tool I've ever encountered to help me make the big choices in life. Because almost everything – all external expectations, all pride, all fear of embarrassment or failure – these things just fall away in the face of death, leaving only what is truly important. Remembering that you are going to die is the best way I know to avoid the trap of thinking you have something to lose. You are already naked. There is no reason not to follow your heart.

No one wants to die. Even people who want to go to heaven don't want to die to get there. And yet death is the destination we all share. No one has ever escaped it. And that is as it should be, because Death is very likely the single best invention of Life. It is Life's change agent. It clears out the old to make way for the new. Right now the new is you, but someday not too long from now, you will gradually become the old and be cleared away.

Your time is limited, so don't waste it living someone else's life. Don't be trapped by dogma – which is living with the results of other people's thinking. Don't let the noise of others' opinions drown out your own inner voice. And most important, have the courage to follow your heart and intuition. They somehow already know what you truly want to become. Everything else is secondary."

I am doing my best to live as Jobs recommends.

Yalom also recommends "...*living an authentic life of engagement, connectivity, meaning, and self-fulfillment...*" I'm doing my best to live an authentic life by being a compassionate friend, a loving mother and grandmother, and by creating as many "ripples" as I can. I hope to have no more regrets. This is what we should all do because death comes to all of us and we never know when.

Letter To My 91 Year-Old Mother About Death & Dying

Dear Mom,

Recently you told me you have been feeling depressed because so many of your friends and family are dying, and this causes you to think about your own death. Having a Stage IV cancer diagnosis, I too have been depressed thinking about my sooner-than-expected death. However, I no longer feel that way; I feel at peace about death and dying. Why?

I've been reading Buddhist principles and finding much comfort in their view of death. Death is the one certainty of life; we will all die (and we never know when). Rather than denying death, Buddhists believe that accepting and even embracing death helps us to live a more meaningful and fulfilling life. If we accept that we will die at some point, we are more likely to enjoy the present moment and make the most of each day; we are more likely to focus on what's most important to us and live accordingly. This is how I try to live.

It became crystal clear to me, when I got my diagnosis, that what's most important to me are my family and friends – my relationships – so I do my best to create more positive memories (especially with my three grandchildren). I also want to feel that I have made a positive difference in the world, so I continue to do what I can to help others (writing this blog is one way I do that; life coaching is another way). I also focus on the contributions I've made in the past that I'm proud of, and I try to be grateful every day for all the gifts in my life.

Buddhists also believe in reincarnation. I'm not sure I believe in this, but none of us knows for certain what happens after we die. A startling number of people who have survived a near-death experience have been left with a conviction that life continues after death. There seems to be a core experience from all who have been near death: they feel enveloped in light and love; they feel at peace, without pain or fear; some see dead loved ones welcoming them; most do a life-review. Buddhists believe that the moment of death is the moment of profound transformation and spiritual awakening. I find comfort in all this, don't you?

*The central message that near-death experiencers bring back from their encounters with death is that the essential and most important qualities in life are love, knowledge, compassion, and wisdom. And **love conquers all**. So if we live each day seeking happiness, finding wisdom, being mindful and grateful and loving and compassionate, we will hopefully die at peace with few regrets. I'm doing my best to live this way.*

After I'm gone I hope that my friends and family will have fond memories of me; I hope that they will think that I enriched their life in some way. I want you to know that you have enriched my life in so many ways: you've shown me how to take risks, to be unattached to "stuff", to be a life-long learner, to take a stand for things I believe in, to question authority. You exposed me to different cultures and countries. You were an inspiring role model: someone who believed she could do anything she put her mind to, and did – getting your college degree in your 50's, being a social director on a cruise ship, traveling the world, being a successful writer and speaker, etc. I want you to know that some part of you will always be within me; you have created many "ripples" of influence that have profoundly affected me and, I'm sure, many others whose lives you have touched.

I hope that this letter has eased your depression a bit and that you feel less anxious and fearful about facing death. I hope, instead, that you will focus on all you have given to me and to your family and friends, because that is what I focus on. Know that you have lived a rich and fascinating life, filled with adventure and meaning.

With much love, Laurie

Conclusion

This book is only the beginning. I will continue to post my lung cancer journey at www.ingearcoaching.com/blog, and I do hope that people will continue to read it for years to come. But, for now, I wanted to document the first five years of my journey.

The posts are meant to be *informative...* providing facts and figures and resources... as well as *personal...* sharing my fears and challenges and coping strategies. My goal is to enrich and enhance the lives of others; my hope is to leave a lasting legacy. If this book does that, I've been successful.

Dr. Eben Alexander, in his book, <u>Proof of Heaven</u>, said that the most important message he got from his near-death experience was that **love** is the basis of everything. I agree with him. He was told: *"Love is the only thing that truly matters... we are loved. Love is not some abstract, hard-to-fathom kind of love, but the day-to-day kind that everyone knows – the kind of love we feel when we look at our spouse and our children, or even our animals. In its purest and most powerful form, this love is not jealous or selfish, but unconditional. This is the reality of realities, the incomprehensibly glorious truth of truths that lives and breathes at the core of everything that exists or that ever will exist, and no remotely accurate understanding of who and what we are can be achieved by anyone who does not know it, and embody it in all of their actions."*

Being diagnosed with lung cancer made me focus on what matters most in my life: my love for my family and friends and the love I receive from them. With love I can face cancer and life's other challenges with less fear and more peace; I can be happy. That's what life is all about.

"Love – it surrounds every being and extends slowly to embrace all that shall be." ~ Khalil Gibran

Acknowledgments

So many people have supported me in my cancer journey as I'm *Dancing Through Cancer*. Words are inadequate in expressing my appreciation, but here is a list (not in any particular order) of all who have cared for me along the way.

Thanks to my son, *Scott*, and daughter-in-law, *Lisa*, and my grandchildren, *Madison, Taylor,* and *Jack,* for taking care of me at their house (and giving me their bed) during my two-month lung surgery recuperation and, later, recovering from chemotherapy infusions. Thank you for being there at the hospital during and after surgery, and later.

Thanks to my other son, *Derek,* for coming to the hospital post surgery (and wanting to camp out there with me!), and for staying with me after a chemotherapy infusion. I will always remember our fabulous trip to Mexico together, while celebrating my being in remission. I'm especially appreciative of your moving to Gloucester to be closer to me during this challenging time in my life. I've cherished our time together.

A special thanks to *Francine,* my private nurse friend, who has dedicated herself to being my personal medical advocate. She drives down from Vermont to go with me to my medical appointments; this means I'm never alone to hear bad (or good) news. Francine also goes with me to as many Zydeco dances as we can arrange; she's my dancing buddy as I'm *Dancing Through Cancer!*

Thanks to my women's group: *Claudia Schweitzer* who set up the schedules for doctor appointments, weekend infusion recoveries, home visits; *Sandy Dahl* who went with me to my breast surgery (lumpectomy); *Michele Harrison* who accompanied me to an MRI procedure (where we had a bit of an amusing incident!) and who let me live at her house many nights; *Lizzie Barron* who, along with her husband, *Billy,* also took care of me in their home many, many nights; and *Pat Burke* who never forgets to call or write encouragement. I thank them all for the powerful healing circle they gave me, for all the phone calls/emails/cards, and for the focused support during our group sessions.

Additional thanks go to *Gail Burchard,* who nursed me over a "chemo" weekend and who also stayed to care for me post lumpectomy. More thanks go to *Laila O'Keeffe* who has accompanied me to many MRI appointments, as has *Lee Cunningham.* And thanks to *Lee* and her husband, *John,* for the many post-chemo healing sailing trips to Maine!

Thanks to *Barbara Shesky* who flew up from Georgia to care for me during SRS.

Many thanks go to *Grace Durfee* who gifted me Reiki treatments, both distant and in-person, and for training me to do Reiki on myself.

Thanks go to *Margi Green* for all the massages (and stretches) she has given me to reduce blockages. And many thanks to *Lacey D'Amico* for figuring out how to style my new hairdo; and more thanks to *Alexi Ruvolo* for keeping away the painful (toe nail) paronykias with her pedicures.

Thanks to all my other friends and family who continue to support me through calls and emails and home visits: *Ginny O'Brien, Lucille Homcy, Christina & Warren Brodie, Paul & Janet Butler, Nancy & Jay Smith, Bob & Sherrie Cutler, Nancy*

& *Gordon Massingham, Peter & Polly Reed,* and special thanks go to *Mary & Dave Browne,* my landlords, who have rented me my place in paradise on earth.

A big thanks goes to my financial advisors who have helped me create a financial plan that allows me to live a full and happy life: *Carl Alviti* and *Adam Rogers.* Thank you for all your personalized and caring service.

To *Liza,* my niece who is the daughter I always wanted; we've shared lots of adventures (Macchu Pichu! Costa Rica...). Thanks for all your loving kindness over the years.

Thanks to *Cal,* my nephew, and wife *Monica* for making the effort to spend Christmas with our family when I couldn't travel post surgery and post chemo; and thanks for taking me skiing.

Thanks to *Samantha,* my other niece, for knitting me a lovely healing shawl.

Thanks to my sister, *Ceci,* who is my greatest teacher of patience, humility, compassion, and finding unconditional love.

Thanks to my mother, *Rhoda,* who always encouraged me to *write it all down!* She is my other great teacher!

Thanks to *Mickey,* my other mother, who has been there for me since I was a teenager. I love my home-away-from home on her farm. Thank you for all the horseback riding over the years!

And I can't thank enough my special cousin (my second sister), *Chrissy,* for the many, many nights at her house in La Jolla, and for always being willing to listen to me vent; we've had some amazing adventures together over the years.

Thanks to cousin, *Cinda,* for all her wise advice; and thanks to cousin *Betsy,* for all her support of my mother.

I'd like to also acknowledge my *Dad* and my *Brother,* who I am sure would be thankful NOT to be reading this book. I'm glad I spared them the fears and concerns of my diagnosis. Although I think my brother would have been my best nurse!

Thanks, especially, to my doctors for keeping me alive! *Dr. Michael Lanuti,* my lung surgeon; *Dr. Jennifer Temel,* my main oncologist, whose expertise and cheerfulness are always so appreciated and valued; *Dr. Andrew Lane,* the oncology Fellow who treated me for over three years, who always had unlimited time for me, and who would call me back immediately with any of my concerns. I miss him!; *Dr. Martin Cutler* who has doggedly and cheerily helped me manage all my eye problems.

Thanks to *Fernando,* my personal doctor, who was there for me in so many ways when I needed him.

And, of course, thanks go to *MJ Schwader,* my writing coach and editor, who helped me make this book happen. I hope it's just the beginning of many more books to come.

And many thanks go to all the people who have responded to my *Carepages* and my blog – your support and caring have always boosted my spirits; you are all amazing.

If I have forgotten to thank anyone else, please forgive me. We'll blame it on chemo-brain! I still love you.

Offering Cancer Coaching

More and more hospitals and clinics are hiring life coaches to provide wellness coaching for cancer patients. Life coaching has been around for several decades, but has recently gained more prominence in the cancer community. This arose out of a growing awareness – especially among patients themselves – that treatment often didn't focus on the whole person, but rather on the disease.

In a recent research study, 30 cancer patients participated in wellness coaching over a three-month period. Published by *The International Journal of Interdisciplinary Social Sciences*, the results showed various improvements, including decreased depression and anxiety, increased physical activity, better motivation, and a healthier diet. Other studies have indicated coaches can help patients communicate better with their doctors, make better health care choices, manage transitions, and maintain better relationships with family and friends. Life and wellness coaches provide cancer patients with support and guidance in the following areas: relationships, nutrition, exercise, work, and stress management. Coaches can help patients adjust to living their "new normal" life, managing all the changes and losses related to cancer. Alternatively, coaches can help patients face and deal with the very real prospect of death and dying.

Life coaching assists people in identifying, then prioritizing, specific goals, then taking action to reach those goals faster and with greater ease, providing a structure and process that holds the client accountable for the chosen actions. In addition, cancer coaching supports the client in dealing with all the challenges related to living with cancer.

As a cancer survivor and certified life coach I hope to coach other cancer survivors and their caretakers. I will support clients during their cancer journey by helping them:

- deal with hearing the cancer diagnosis for the first time.

- accept receiving negative results from follow-up diagnostic procedures.

- celebrate positive results from follow-up diagnostic procedures.

- manage treatment side effects.

- manage change; live in transition.

- learn to live with all the losses associated with cancer treatments.

- explore new options; making new choices.

- take risks for personal growth.

- make difficult decisions.

- set realistic goals for the future.

- learn to lead a healthier life style through proper nutrition, exercise, and stress management.

- provide helpful tools, resources, and referrals, as needed.

- help reframe beliefs and offer different perspectives and ideas.

- create a nurturing support system; minimize unsupportive behaviors.

- set boundaries necessary for personal care.

- develop an attitude of gratitude.

• face and plan for the end of life.

Most of all… I will help clients learn to live well in their "new normal" life.

My goal is to guide clients through their cancer journey by empowering them, providing emotional support while helping them build their strength and develop courage to face all their challenges. I want to help clients be proactive in their own health care by sharing resources, tools, and information that I have found helpful in my journey. I will be a listening ear, a trusted friend, an encouraging and supportive partner, and a fellow traveler on this difficult cancer journey.

I offer complimentary phone consultations. For more information, go to www.ingearcoaching.com. To contact me, email ingear@comcast.net or call 617-947-7430.

Resources

Recommended Books

Proof of Heaven: A Neurosurgeon's Journey into the Afterlife, by Eben Alexander, M.D. After his NDE (near death experience), Dr. Alexander is convinced that death is not the end of personal existence, but a transition into an afterlife.

Staring at the Sun: Overcoming the Terror of Death, by Irvin Yalom.

On Death & Dying, by Elizabeth Kubler-Ross

When Things Fall Apart: Heart Advice for Difficult Times, by Pema Chodron.

The Portable Coach: The 28 Principles of Attraction, by Thomas Leonard.

Home Before Dark: A Family Portrait of Cancer and Healing, by David, Kate, Michael, & Sam Treadway

The Starch Solution, by John McDougall. In his new book, McDougall makes it crystal clear, with vast supportive research, that a plant-based diet is the only way to live healthy. The Starch Solution Recipe book is also available.

The China Study by T. Colin Campbell. Through his groundbreaking research, Campbell shows the link between dairy and cancer, and other diseases.

Crazy, Sexy Cancer by Kris Carr. Carr tells her personal story of surviving an extremely rare sarcoma called epithelioid hemangioendothelioma (EHE) by eating only a plant-based diet. She was only given a few months to live, yet nine years later, she is alive and well. Crazy, Sexy Diet and Crazy, Sexy Kitchen give us excellent recipes for a plant-based diet.

Anti-Cancer: A New Way of Life by Dr. Servan-Schreiber, M.D. Diagnosed with brain cancer, Dr. Servan-Schreiber extended his life by years by mostly following a plant-based diet.

Healing with the Mind's Eye by Dr. Michael Samuels. This book shows how to use guided imagery to heal the body, mind, and spirit.

The Human Side of Cancer: Living with Hope, Coping with Uncertainty, by Jimmie Holland & Sheldon Lewis.

Voices of Lung Cancer: The Healing Companion – Stories for Courage, Comfort, and Strength by The Healing Project and Epath Merhuen.

Perspectives of a Flying Elephant: My First Year in the Land of Lung Junk, by Teri Simon. This book is a chronicle of one woman's first year of living with lung cancer. It is told in a series of blog posts that are frank, warm, humor-infused, and, most of all, full of hope. (See also Teri's book: My Second Year in the Land of Lung Junk.) Sadly, Teri died at the end of her third year battling lung cancer.

Living with Lung Cancer: My Journey, by Thomas Cappiello.

The Engine 2 Diet by Rip Esselstyn. Esselstyn wrote this book because of the success he and his fire-fighting buddies had in drastically reducing their cholesterol levels by incorporating a plant-based diet.

The Blood Sugar Solution: The Ultra-Healthy Program for Losing Weight, Preventing Disease, and Feeling Great Now, by Mark Hyman.

The Cancer Survivor's Guide: Foods that Help you Fight Back, by Neal Barnard.

Diet for a Small Planet by Frances Moore Lappe. Let's not forget the one who started the plant-based diet conversation.

Dr. Nicholas Gonzales, of New York, has also had a lot of success with his treatment protocol, mostly based on a healthy diet of fruits, vegetables, and plant foods. You can read more about him in Suzanne Somers' book, Knockout: Interviews with Doctors who are Curing Cancer and How to Prevent it in the First Place.

Recommended Films

Dr. Gerson, also mentioned in Suzanne Somers' book, claimed he cured cancer back in the 1940's. The Gerson Clinic continues to cure cancer patients today by using a strict nutritional therapy regime. For more information about the Gerson clinic, watch "The Gerson Miracle" or "The Beautiful Truth."

"Cut, Poison, Burn" is a shocking documentary on the dangerous shortcomings of the Western medicine approach to cancer treatment. The film shows how alternative medical treatments (that work!) are actively blocked by large pharmaceutical companies. *We are a wealth society, not a health society.*

"Fat, Sick, and Nearly Dead" relates the story of two very over-weight men (350 - 430 lbs.) who lose weight (to 200+ lbs.) and become very healthy by juicing with green plants and fruits.

"Food Matters" is a ground-breaking documentary that uncovers the trillion dollar worldwide "sickness industry" and exposes a growing body of scientific evidence proving that nutritional therapy can be more effective, more economical, less harmful, and less invasive than most conventional medical treatments.

"Hungry for Change" is a documentary that empowers and provides practical and realistic solutions to healthy nutrition.

"Forks Over Knives" is a documentary that examines the profound claim that most, if not all, of the degenerative diseases that afflict us can be controlled, or even reversed, by rejecting animal-based and processed foods.

"Food, Inc" shows how our cattle and chickens are raised: squished in a feed lot or a window-less building, fed only corn, ingested with antibiotics and steroids.

"Fast Food Nation" shows how we are all affected by the fast food industry and the real and disturbing flaws that exist in meatpacking plants.

"The Future of Food" documents what is currently going on with the food supply in the U.S., which is dominated by Monsanto.

"How to Cook Your Life" shows how Buddhism and cooking unite.

"Supersize Me" is the story of a man who eats nothing but McDonald's food for months and almost kills himself.

"Vegucated" is a guerrilla-style documentary that follows three meat and cheese loving New Yorkers who agree to adopt a vegan diet for six weeks to learn what it's all about. Shockingly exposed are the methods by which animals and chickens are slaughtered for market.

"Fresh" points out the value of eating fresh fruits and vegetables as often as possible.

"Sugar: The Bitter Truth" is a movie about the dangers of sugar; search for it on *YouTube*.

Magazines

"Nutrition Action Newsletter" for excellent, up-to-date information on healthy eating, along with some great recipes.

"Cure" - free to cancer patients.

Recommended Websites

Beatcancer.org

Inspire.com/groups/cancer-treatment

Kriscarr.com

Curetoday.com

Facing-cancer.org

Freetobreathe.com

Johnbagnulo.com

Lungcanceralliance.org

Events.lungevity.org

Canceradvocacy.org

Nationallungcancerpartnership.org

Unitingagainslungcancer.org

Thecancerjourney.com

Eternea.org

Activesurvivor.org

Teamsurvivor.org

Carepages.com (lauriegeary2008)

Laurie's Other Publications

Gear Up With Games! *Games & Initiatives For Networking, Energizing, Team-Building... and just plain Fun!* This Booklet is filled with over 100 experiential games and activities drawn from Laurie's years of experience as an Outward Bound Instructor.

Gear Up For Success! *Create the Life You Want Through Responsible Risk-Taking.* This workbook is filled with articles, top tens, exercises, quotes/poems, and models to give a boost to personal and professional growth through responsible risk-taking.

A Guide to Getting It: Self-Esteem - *Ideas and Tools from Life and Business Coaches to Help You Live Your Life's Dreams,* edited by MJ Schwader. The book includes 12 chapters written by 12 different coaches on ways to develop self-awareness in order to build self-esteem. Laurie's chapter "Risk-Taking and Building Self-Esteem" presents her awesome *8-A Model* for taking responsible risks that lead to personal growth.

Gear Up For Success with Assertiveness Training! (an eCourse)

Laurie has many, many newsletters, written weekly for two years on her website: www.ingearcoaching.com.

To read more specific medical details of Laurie's cancer journey, go to www.carepages.com and search for lauriegeary2008.

About Laurie Riddell Geary

Laurie grew up in La Jolla, California, where she spent most of her time at the beach – swimming and watching surfers. She also loved to spend time at her aunt's ranch in Alpine where she would ride horses and climb rocks.

Besides California, she has lived in Mexico, Spain, Germany, Puerto Rico, Argentina, Virginia, Rhode Island, New Hampshire, and now Massachusetts. She has traveled to China, Southeast Asia, Europe, South America, the Dominican Republic, Costa Rica, Morocco, Hawaii, Australia, and New Zealand.

Laurie attended Mary Washington College, then graduated from the University of Virginia with a B.S. in Education. Later she attended Boston University, graduating with an M.Ed. (Masters in Psychological Education). Much later she became a Professional Certified Life Coach (PCC).

Professionally she has taught high school English and Spanish and been a guidance counselor. For years she was an instructor for Outward Bound Professional Programs and for the Appalachian Mountain Club's Leadership School; she has been a career transition specialist for Lee Hecht Harrison and Right Management; she continues to be an on-line instructor for the Teacher Education Institute. She is a consultant and trainer who has developed many diverse programs and workshops over the years. Laurie has been a professional life coach for almost 20 years, helping people in life/career transition; now she wants to use her skills and experience to coach those dealing with cancer. Bi-lingual, she has taught and consulted in Spanish.

Besides dancing, Laurie loves to ski, hike, bike, kayak, windsurf, and sail.

Now happily single, Laurie was married for 28 years. She has two sons and three grandchildren with whom she tries to spend as much time as possible.

She lives in Gloucester, Massachusetts, overlooking the ocean where she has time to write and reflect and *dance through cancer.*

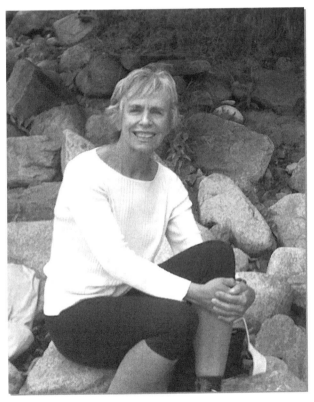

Laurie Riddell Geary

Made in the USA
Middletown, DE
06 April 2016